# "Muscle Testing"

## Complete Nonsense?

## Or the Basis for Real Health Care?

## by

## Serafino Amoroso

Bloomington, IN    authorHOUSE™    Milton Keynes, UK

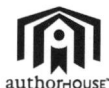

*AuthorHouse™*
*1663 Liberty Drive, Suite 200*
*Bloomington, IN 47403*
*www.authorhouse.com*
*Phone: 1-800-839-8640*

*AuthorHouse™ UK Ltd.*
*500 Avebury Boulevard*
*Central Milton Keynes, MK9 2BE*
*www.authorhouse.co.uk*
*Phone: 08001974150*

*This book is a work of non-fiction. Unless otherwise noted, the author and the publisher make no explicit guarantees as to the accuracy of the information contained in this book and in some cases, names of people and places have been altered to protect their privacy.*

*First published by AuthorHouse 2/27/2006*

*ISBN: 1-4208-6772-5 (sc)*

*Library of Congress Control Number: 2005905704*

*Printed in the United States of America*
*Bloomington, Indiana*

*This book is printed on acid-free paper.*

## Preliminary Remark

I put the words *muscle testing* in the title in quotes because although that's what this topic is commonly called, I don't care for the term, at least not as applied to what I'll be discussing which has little to do with the testing of muscles themselves. Also, the only muscles I'll be using are certain muscles in the upper part of the arm and shoulder (those of the deltoid family), and I'll be *using* these to test a wide variety of other factors but not the muscles themselves. The term "kinesiological testing" is also commonly used for what I'll be discussing, but this is to redefine the term from its traditional use as applying to a medical discipline having nothing to do with our subject.[1] *Applied Kinesiology* is a related topic that also uses muscles for testing but this is not our topic. I'll be using the term "muscle-response testing" which is perhaps a little more accurate for our purposes.

---

1. For information on the medical discipline, see for example: *Muscles: Testing and Function* by Kenndle and Kenndle. Williams & Wilkins, 2nd Edition, 1971.

# Section 1: A Little History and a Little Orientation

*"The universe is not to be narrowed down to the limits of our understanding ... but our understanding must be stretched and enlarged to take in the image of the universe as it is discovered."*

*Francis Bacon*

### How did it all start for me?

It was at a seminar in New York City in a hotel in Gramercy Park around 1990 that I first saw a demonstration of a muscle-response test and my belief system was turned on its head. The demonstration was given by Dr. Jose Rodriguez DC, who was one of the first diplomates of *Applied Kinesiology*. I was really impressed, and I could see there was so much more to reality than I could have imagined. I was a beginning student at the time at a small naturopathic school, and since that time as I went on with my education, many of my teachers used muscle-response testing as the central tool relating to what they were teaching: Dr. Herb Anderson's monthly lectures in Stanford Connecticut on *Applied Kinesiology*; Dr. Eugene Charles' hundred-hour professional course on *Applied Kinesiology*; Dr. John Thie and his *Touch for Health*; Dr. John Diamond's lectures on applications of muscle-response testing into the domain of emotional health; Dr. D.A. Versendaal's seminars on his *Contact Reflex Analysis*; Dr. Dan Gole's seminars on the application of muscle-response testing to dentistry; Dr. Scott Walker's NET (*Neuro-Emotional Technique®*); Dr. Wendell Whitman's courses on various topics in the health sciences many of which used muscle-response testing; and finally my friend Dr. Walter Melnicke who taught me most about muscle-response testing. There were other teachers at weekend seminars as well whose names I've forgotten.

With all of this, I've come to see very clearly that there is much of great importance that goes beyond the boundaries of mainstream science, even beyond the boundaries of our Western, materialistic

1

beliefs. One of my purposes in writing this book is help you come to the same conclusion.

As far as I know, what I'll be discussing is not taught at any conventional school in this country, or in any other country for that matter. All the instruction I mentioned above was outside of mainstream academia.

I should also say that it is certain that none of the teachers mentioned above will agree with everything I've written in this book. Certainly much of what I've written I've learned from them, but anything said here that is not correct should be attributed to me alone. The only blame they deserve is for getting me intensely interested in this work.

I've used muscle-response testing in my practice now for over twelve years. In the early days, not surprisingly, none of my new clients had ever seen muscle-response testing and for most it seemed too crazy to be believed and few would return after the first office visit. Now it's still difficult for many of my clients to believe, but it's not at all unusual for new clients to have already seen or even experienced muscle-response testing. If you're new to this it will probably be difficult for you also not to see this as all nonsense. Even if you're not seeing this for the first time and you're already a believer, I'm sure much of what I'll be describing here will also be new to you.

**Is it making its way to the mainstream?**

A very conventional dentist and friend of mine told me recently that at a seminar he had just attended (dentists are required to attend seminars on a regular basis to keep their licenses) the speaker who was from a dental school associated with a major university in the Boston area *demonstrated muscle-response testing*!

On national television recently, Dr. Wayne Dyer told a story about his teenaged son and some annoying music the son had been listening to. Dr. Dyer just held the CD near his son and using muscle-response testing the son was unable to hold up his arm!

There is precedent for the boundaries of reality of conventional belief to grow. Thirty years ago the boundaries in the US certainly did not include acupuncture. Mirium Lee tells in her book *Reflections of a Senior Acupuncturist* of her arrest in California in 1970 for doing some strange therapy with needles. Today acupuncture is generally accepted all over the US.

## What do I hope to accomplish here?

My purpose here is to introduce you the reader to muscle-response testing and to some of its applications. This is a very large topic so please look upon this as if I'm taking you on a guided tour and showing you some of the highlights. My intention here is certainly not to teach you how to do this work, however, I'm sure there will be some demonstrations I'll be showing you that you'll be unable to avoid trying. Fortunately, there are some simple tests you should be able to do that can also be really useful. But for the most part, much of what I'll be describing should be done only by a professional health care provider properly trained to do this work. This is not a book intended to train anyone but I certainly hope it will interest some health care professionals to investigate the topic further. I will be giving some sources for this purpose later.

If what I'm showing you is correct, then not only should it be of considerable interest, but I believe it should be the basis of a health care system that will really be concerned with *health* care and can be an answer to the huge costs of our current system of *sickness care* that is bankrupting the country and not making us any healthier.

Finally, there is the question of *how* does all this work. I'm certain that no one as yet has the definitive answer to this question; I can only give you opinions that I've heard from others and some of my own. I'll do this as we move along.

## Applied Kinesiology and Muscle-Response Testing

So where did muscle-response testing come from? How did all of this get started? It was discovered by Dr. George Goodheart DC in the 1960's who went on to develop the field of *Applied Kinesiology* (AK) which is totally based on muscle-response testing. It's amazing to me how such a simple phenomenon had apparently gone unknown throughout human history. Of course the testing of muscles as might be done by a physical therapist has been part of medicine before the 1960's, probably going back into prehistory, but what we will be discussing here has no relation to this.

There are at least two kinds of muscle-response testing. The first kind which will *not* be discussed in this book is based on the fundamental premise that there's an association between muscles and organs. For example, the pectoralis sternum (which are muscles in your chest) are related to the liver, the sartorius (muscles in the legs) to the adrenals, the fascia lata (in the outer thigh) to the large intestines, and so forth. A major discovery by Dr. Goodheart was *if an organ had some significant dysfunction the corresponding muscle would test weak.* Much of the testing done in AK therefore involves isolating specific muscles for testing. As I said, we will not be discussing this kind of testing in this book.[1] The second kind of muscle-response testing uses muscles as *indicators,* as a general means of "communicating with the body," and except for convenience, it doesn't matter what muscle is used. This is using muscle-response testing in a very different manner, and this manner of testing will be used throughout this book. Applied Kinesiology actually makes use of both of these methods of testing.

Before we leave the muscle-organ relationship, how difficult is it to believe that there is a relation of muscles to organs? Many reject this along with all else about AK as nonsense, but they should at least consider this: It's part of mainstream embryonic science that as the fetus develops, muscles and organs develop sharing nerve and venous systems. So should the correspondence between muscles and organs experienced by muscle-response testing in AK be so surprising? Beyond even this, just witness an experienced AK practitioner and how can you not believe your eyes?[2]

# Endnotes

1. See e.g., the book by Walther: Applied Kinesiology: Synopsis. SDC Systems DC, 275 West Abriendo Aveenue, Pueblo, Colorado 81004.

2. Groucho Marx caught in bed with another woman by his wife said "Who are you going to believe, me or your eyes?"

# Section 2: An Introduction to the Technique

## An Idealized Muscle-Response Test

Now let's take our first look at a muscle-response test. Assume there's a person that's agreed to be the subject of the test. I ask the person if there is any physical problem with his arms or shoulders. If there is none I then ask the person to hold out an arm horizontally to the side (say the right arm)[1], and with my left hand I put some downward pressure just above the person's wrist and the arm tests strong, that is, I can't easily push it down. Somewhat like a piano key, as I put pressure on the arm it feels as if I hit a bottom, we call it "feeling a locking of the muscle." Now I perform some test, let's say I point to an organ reflex point (I'll soon be explaining what this means and describing many other kinds of tests) and if the arm can still take the same downward pressure as before and still stay up, that is, I still feel the locking, then the test is *negative*. This might mean a weakness in the organ associated with the reflex point was not found. If on the other hand the arm drops; the person is unable to hold up the arm; I can pull it down easily, then the test is *positive*[2]. This could mean, for example, that an organ weakness that needs attention has been found.[3] Sometimes the positive outcome of such a test is dramatic in the sense that the subject's arm drops as if it went paralyzed. This is the response from a positive test we would like from everyone, but at times a test result is not so clear.

## A Less Idealized Muscle-Response Test

*"As you work on the blockages the person's arm will drop more dramatically. I like to see the arm really drop!"*

*D.A.Versendaal.*

Of course by applying a great deal of pressure one can force almost any arm to drop. It should be made clear to the subject new to all this that a muscle-response test is not an arm-wrestling contest, the practitioner is just feeling to see if the arm can "lock" or not. When the person can't lock the muscle, it is near impossible to resist the arm going down. Any practitioner using muscle-response testing experiences a wide variety of responses from different individuals. Some persons will be amazingly testable and the response is absolutely clear. Then there will be persons testable but the response will not be as clear as you might wish. Some will need a lot of pressure and some very little. There will also be persons that seem impossible to test giving no response at all; either the arm is always strong or always weak. I'll later discuss some procedures that I would try if I'm faced with this situation.[4]

In the description above, I used the person's (right) arm as a so-called "indicator." In fact, just about any muscle of the body can be used although to me none are usually as convenient as the arm. The "o-ring" formed by touching a thumb and pointer finger is used by some practitioners, the test being to try to pull the fingers apart. Isolating a muscle in a leg and using it as indicator is often used, especially in AK

**You pushed harder!**

It is common when a person first experiences muscle-response testing to feel their response was not different when it was supposed to be weak from when it was supposed to be strong. They will often say "you pushed harder the second time." Or "You pushed differently the second time." Or better: "Try that again." They often react this way no matter how clear the response. Why is this so? It's really not difficult to see why. There is nothing in their belief system to explain what is happening except that you must have pushed harder when the arm went down. It's the only explanation they have. With repeated experience they usually (almost always) come to believe it does work (you didn't actually push harder).

Any physical movement that takes place in the human body involves a muscle or a group of muscles tightening while complementary muscles loosen. Then making the opposite motion the muscles that tightened now loosen and the ones that loosened tighten. This goes on smoothly, automatically and continuously without any conscious thought. The loosening and tightening of muscles is one of the most common features of all human (and animal) life. This facility must certainly be involved in muscle-response testing.

## Some Terminology

In professional terminology, the muscle being used during a test is called the *indicator*. Here in this book the indicator will always be a deltoid muscle (they're the muscles located where the arms connect to the shoulders); we will always use an arm for testing. When during a test the arm drops, the more technical description is to say *the indicator is inhibited,* and if the arm does not drop *the indicator is facilitated.* In what follows we will be less formal and just say *"the arm is strong,"* or *"the arm remains strong"* or *the arm "goes weak"* or *"the arm drops".*

Interpreting the outcome of a muscle-response test as *positive* if the arm drops or *negative* if the arm remains strong will not always be correct. In different situations the opposite may be the case. An arm going weak can also mean either a "yes" or a "no" or even something besides a yes or no.

## Can anyone do muscle-response testing?

If the question is changed slightly and I'm asked if anyone can learn to do muscle-response testing, I'd like to think the answer would be yes, but I'm afraid I have to give a qualified No! I haven't done any research on this but I think a person very prejudiced against this, thinking it nonsense, will not be able to get a response. I'll have more to say later on this topic. The section on *Problems,* presented later, will also be relevant to this question.

For the professional healthcare practitioner wishing to look further into all this, there is no substitute to taking a professional seminar or a course of instruction where muscle-response testing is used and taught. My hope is that some day every chiropractor will study and become proficient in Applied Kinesiology which I believe has the potential to raise the profession of Chiropractic to a much higher level of excellence than it has even now. Professional courses are offered regularly through *the International College of Applied Kinesiology.*[5]

## A Simple Example of a Muscle-Response Test

Here's a simple but very important example of a muscle-response test: Visualize a person who is the subject of the test standing in front of me. I ask the person to extend say the left arm horizontally out to the side. I then put my right hand on the person's wrist of the extended arm and ask the subject to match the pressure I'm going to use. I then slowly put some downward pressure feeling how the person can resist the pressure. Let's assume the person can resist easily, that is, the muscles holding up the arm feel strong to me. Now with the pointer finger of my left hand I touch the top of the subject's nose (the area between the eyes) and simultaneously repeat the pressure on the extended arm. The arm now drops, the person being unable to hold it up.

Actually I perform this test on every person at the start of every office visit. I call this the "battery test." I use it to see if I can "communicate" with this person.[6] The communication I'm referring to is of course not the usual verbal communication between us but rather the one that takes place through the muscle-response procedures.

# Endnotes

1. I've never noticed a difference between using the right or left arm, unless of course one arm has a physical weakness. Dr. Melnicke prefers using the person's left arm.

2. There will be some exceptions to the interpretation of positive and negative.

3. The example is actually describing an alternative way of testing for organ weakness, alternative from the muscle-isolating technique used in AK mentioned above.

4. This is actually a large topic that we plan to document elsewhere.

5. See Appendix E

6. I personally don't actually touch the top of the subject's nose; it's enough for me to just point to it.

# Section 3: Some Demonstrations

As we go through different demonstrations, I'll offer some more or less feasible explanations for the behavior being described. I offer these without necessarily claiming total belief in what I'm saying. I'm also not claiming that I don't believe what I'm saying. What I'm trying to say is they are put forth as hypotheses. I guess this is the way science has always developed; phenomena are observed and theories are put forth. As further phenomena are observed the theories are strengthened, modified or perhaps discarded for new ones.

Here is one hypothesis: There is an energy emanating out from the fingers (this can actually be verified e.g. by Kirlian photography[1]), and in the above example, this energy is being directed into the lower, frontal part of the brain. There are also acupuncture points in the immediate area of the dip at the top of the nose between the eyes, and this energy is interacting with these.

**The Meridian/Acupuncture System of the Body**

In preparation for our next demonstration I should say a few words about the Chinese meridian/acupuncture system. In classical Chinese medicine, it is believed that there are two different, but both absolutely necessary ways the human body is nourished.[2] One of these is *physical nourishment* involving substances such as food, enzymes, herbs, water, oxygen, sunlight, etc. The second of these is not part of Western tradition and involves what the Chinese call *Qi* (pronounced "chee"). Qi can be thought of as an energy that is breathed into the body from the atmosphere and then circulates throughout the body through very specific pathways giving life and energy to our organs and all other parts of our bodies. The traditional Chinese physician believes the purpose of acupuncture is to relieve blockages to this flow of energy that can occur at different places in the pathway. Applied Kinesiology, the Neuro-Emotional work of Scott Walker, and the work of John Diamond[3] all make substantial and explicit use of the meridian system and many of its acupuncture points in their use of muscle-response testing. It's my belief that everything I'm discussing in this book has a strong relation to Qi

13

and the meridian/acupuncture system. I also believe I have a lot more to learn about this relationship.

For this next demonstration, I'm using a segment of the meridian system called the *conception vessel* which runs from the lower abdomen straight up the front of the body and "ends"⁴ in the mouth.⁵

**Demonstration 1:** The subject is asked to hold out an arm. We can visualize again the person holding the left arm out horizontally to the side. I ask the person to resist and I then put pressure just above the wrist with my right hand. Let's assume the person easily resists the pressure (the arm locks). Now I move my left hand starting from the area of the person's chin then down the front of the body to the area of the lower abdomen, the movement of my hand down the body is a slow, flowing motion taking about two seconds. It will make no difference to the demonstration if I actually touch the body lightly as I move my hand downward, or if I never actually touch and my hand is a few inches away from the body at all times. Now I immediately repeat the muscle-response test and the person is now unable to resist and the arm falls easily. If I reverse the direction and move my hand from the area of the lower abdomen upward to the chin, the arm will test strong. I can repeat this reversal of direction repeatedly, sweeping up and the arm is strong, sweeping down and it goes weak.⁶

## How is this phenomenon to be explained?

This is put forth for consideration: When the hand is moved downward, it is moving in the reverse direction to the energy flow which is from the lower abdomen upward into the mouth. The energy flow can be visualized as a slow moving stream, and the hand movement in the opposite direction temporarily disrupts the stream of energy flow causing the weakness. Reversing direction, the hand restores the proper direction of flow and the arm tests strong. This same reaction will occur no matter what segment of the meridian system is used. The conception vessel is just convenient for the demonstration.

It probably is the energy emanating from the hand and not the physical hand itself that is disrupting the energy flow.

Is the energy flow outside the body as well as inside? Is your hand disrupting the energy only outside the body? Or is energy flowing out from your fingertips and disrupting the flow of energy inside the body? I don't know the answers to any of these questions.

I often start a lecture with the previous demonstration. There is usually nothing in the belief systems of those in attendance that can explain this and it gets their attention. In fact, there is nothing in Western science that can explain this.

**Demonstration 2:** Here is a test I find very useful and I use it quite often. It was demonstrated by Dr. Herb Anderson some years ago. I test an indicator muscle, say the left arm, and it's strong. I then place my right hand near the subject's abdomen, say in the area near the navel (belly button). I then slowly move my right hand away from the body while simultaneously and continuously testing the indicator. The indicator will usually fall when the right hand is about a foot or so from the body. I believe that the closer to the body the right hand is when the indicator falls, the weaker the body's "aura" or overall energy field of the body.[7] From my experience, the larger this energy field, the more testable the subject will be and probably the more healthy as well. By "more testable" I mean the clearer any test result will be using a muscle-response test.

Here is why I said the last phenomenon demonstrated is so useful. When I find a person is not testable. That is, I can get no response to any test. If I increase the strength of the person's aura, the person often becomes testable! Dr. Anderson showed us how to temporarily increase the strength of a person's aura. You do this by making "figure eights" on the person! Here's what this means: With the subject facing me, while pointing the fingers of my right hand I make large figure eights on the subject. The top of the eight goes across the person's forehead from my right to left as I face the person. My hand then moves down from left to right diagonally across the body. I then make the bottom of the eight across the person's lower abdomen from right to left. I then move diagonally from left to right upward across the body. This is the same way a figure eight is written on a piece of paper. The figure eight's are repeated in a continuous motion three or four times. I don't actually touch any part of the person. My hand is always near but not actually touching the body. After this if you retest the size of the aura it will have increased significantly (i.e., my hand can be moved further from the subject's body before the arm falls). The person is almost always now more testable![8] The increase in the aura by this means is not permanent but does usually last during an office visit. I should mention that making the figure eights in the reverse direction will reduce the size of the person's aura.

### "Can These Last Phenomena be Explained?"

Kirlian photography does show an aura around persons and in fact around all living things. Dr. Anderson's test seems to be confirming this. Of course the existence of the aura is a basic belief in the traditional Eastern medical systems. As far as why the "figure eights" does what it does, I haven't a clue.

# Endnotes

1.. See, for example, Kirlian Photography by John Iovine, Images Publishing, 2000.

2 No doubt it's the same for all animals and perhaps all living things.

3. In my opinion, the most interesting and important research on the interaction of muscle-response testing and the meridian/acupuncture system is being done by Dr. John Diamond MD. A part of this work is documented in his book: *Life Energy*, Paragon House, 1990.

4. The segment *name* is the only thing that "ends." The segment itself is part of a continuous path.

5. For this demonstration we could have used any other segment of the meridian system just as well.

6. Dr. Anderson said he sometimes found persons with this flow direction revered. So far I haven't seen this. Dr. Anderson, for a practical application of something very similar to the last demonstration, would actually touch the body as he traversed the meridian.

7. Dr. Versendaal used a similar test, but he tested how far the energy extended from the finger tips.

8. I know of about thirty other ways of increasing the testability of a subject. This will be documented elsewhere.

# <u>Section 4: Now We're Getting Very Practical</u>

*"If a particular nutritional supplement was given to a patient and the muscle tested strong, it was the right supplement for the patient; if the muscle remained weak, it was not. Other methods of treatment could be similarly evaluated. With Applied Kinesiology, doctors had a really useful therapeutic tool, a system of feedback from the body itself. If they gave a patient the proper treatment, the body would respond immediately as if to say, "Yes, that is what was needed."*

*John Diamond MD from his book: The Body Doesn't Lie*

**Demonstration 3:** Test an indicator muscle and let's say it's strong. Now place a small amount of ordinary table sugar on the person's tongue and retest the arm. It will now test weak. The amount of sugar used can be ridiculously small and the test will come out the same. Sugar will weaken just about anyone!

Here's a line from Louise Gittleman's book: *Lick the Sugar Habit*: "Sugar has been blamed for every known disease, and while these accusations may sound like exaggerations, they are closer to the truth than you might realize." If the arm drops when testing a food, I interpret this as an indication that the body has a strong aversion to what is being tested. This demonstration seems to be verifying the truth of her statement about sugar.[1]

**Demonstration 4:** We can repeat the above test but this time with the person just *holding* some sugar. The test can be performed with some sugar placed in the person's hand, or the person can just be holding a box of sugar, or just holding one of the small packets of sugar that you find on the table at any roadside diner. Just holding the sugar will give the same response as putting some on the tongue! AK insists when testing substances that they actually be tasted. They reject testing by just holding the substance. In my experience what I've just described works perfectly well.

**Demonstration 5:** Have the person *just visualize* holding some sugar (or just visualize holding a box of sugar or holding one of the small packets of sugar) and this also will cause a weakening of the indicator! This also is not part of AK.

**Demonstration 6:** Substituting a can of Coke® (or Pepsi®) in place of the sugar will give the same results.

How about Diet Coke® or Diet Pepsi®? These will weaken the body in the same way. In fact, if the person just holds one of the small packets of NutriSweet® it will weaken the person just as sugar does. "The body" also does not think much of NutriSweet![2]

So what does all this mean? First, the message to me is that the body does not want the sugar, the NutriSweet, the Coke or the Pepsi. Secondly, it's another demonstration that there's more to reality than what most persons think and this "more" can be very useful.

The last demonstrations suggest that various food substances might be tested in this same way, and this turns out to be correct. Those of us who do this work find that white flour products, like the most popular white sandwich breads, weaken most persons. From my experience white flour products are not quite as bad as sugar products, but the majority of persons will test weak with them.[3]

The topic of food intolerances in general is not given much attention by our mainstream medical community, but in my opinion it's an extremely common problem that usually goes undiagnosed. A food allergy manifests very quickly and a person with such a problem usually knows it. Food intolerances are far less easily identified, one reason being that the time between consuming the food and the reactions can be days or even longer. This makes correlation difficult.

Dr. Devi Nambudripad MD has developed a procedure (using muscle-response testing) for finding food intolerances as well as intolerances to other non-food substances. She also developed a desensitization process that from all I hear works very well. [4]

I'll have much more to say about the testing of foods and other nutrients later on.

**The model used to explain what's happening needs to be greatly expanded.**

There's a statement in the wonderful book *The Road Less Traveled* by Dr. Scott Peck that I find fascinating. I'm going to use it as the basis of expanding our model in trying to explain what we've seen so far.

> *"When beginning to work with a new patient I will frequently draw a large circle. Then at the circumference I will draw a small niche. Pointing to the inside of the niche, I say, "That represents your conscious mind. All the rest of the circle, 95 percent or more, represents your unconscious. If you work long enough and hard enough to understand yourself, you will come to discover that this vast part of your mind, of which you now have little awareness, contains riches beyond imagination.""*

Keep in mind that what I'm going to say is only a hypothesis. I offer it only as a possibility.

Here's my thought: You bring a substance like sugar into the aura of a person. *The aura is part of the person* and is used by the subconscious intelligence (where there are "riches beyond imagination") to "feel" the substance and to determine if it is beneficial or not. You might ask "If you hold a bottle with a nutrient inside, how does it know to test the nutrient and not the bottle or not to react to the plastic top."[5] My thought is that your conscious intelligence knows we're interested in the contents of the bottle; why not also your unconscious intelligence? Another thing that should be kept in mind is that every substance gives off a unique vibration (this is accepted by Western science) that possibly can be felt through the aura to the subconscious.

How does one explain testing a substance that you don't actually physically have in your hand, a substance that you are just imagining you have in your hand? It's required that the body has had experience with the substance and reacts based on this knowledge.

Here's a story that is relevant here. I was once giving a talk at a fitness center and I was using a volunteer who was a world-class body builder and had come in fourth in a national body building contest in his country, not the US, but he did speak English fairly well. I should mention before going on that he was reacting to my testing; his arm was going weak during a muscle-response test even though he was physically very strong. I then asked him to imagine holding up a well-known (in our country) loaf of white bread. I tested his arm and it was strong! I was surprised since most tested weak when visualizing this nutritionally-poor bread. It then dawned on me to ask if he knew what the bread was that I was asking him to imagine holding and he said: "I have no idea!" I told him more about the bread and he said: "Oh yes I know what that is." And then he tested weak on the test!

All this should not be so difficult to believe. Don't we all know that animals (especially in the wild) have what we call *instincts* that allow them to know what's good for them and what is not? Why is it so difficult to believe we also have the facility?

Irrespective of all this conjecture, we can do useful work without having any idea as to why what we're doing works. One of my teachers said: "When a patient asks me: How does this work? I answer: It works great!"

Let's move on.

## Therapy Localization

What is now referred to in AK as *therapy localization* was George Goodheart's first major discovery. To me it's no exaggeration when I say it was the greatest discovery relating to the assessment and treatment of health problems ever! Perhaps it's the greatest gift to mankind ever! Therapy localization is very simple and although in itself it's pretty fantastic, it's all that it has led to that makes it so important.

Simply and informally stated:

*Therapy Localization is: If you place your hand near a part of the body where there is some dysfunction, a facilitated muscle, (one that tests strong) an indicator you're using for the test, will go inhibited (will go weak).*

The practitioner placing his or her hand over say the liver (right side in front of the body overlapping the lower ribs) and the arm dropping indicates the liver is in someway in need of help. The same applies to all the other organs as well as other aspects of the body like hair, joints, eyes, etc. A therapy localization that causes a weakening of the indicator signals a problem that needs attention.

From my experience there doesn't seem to be much of a difference between actually touching the body in the area that's being tested or just placing your hand close but not actually touching the body. I usually touch lightly. If the area of the body is a sensitive one, or is one that's not socially acceptable to touch, then instead of the practitioner, the person being tested can do the touching and everything works just as well. In fact, the person being tested can always do the touching instead of the practitioner.

Therapy localization is such an important discovery, yet it's so utterly simple. When you see it applied later in the different contexts, you should see why I believe it's so important.

As an example, imagine I'm testing an indicator arm and it's strong. With my other hand I press my fingers lightly into the area just below rib cage in the center of the body[6] and simultaneously retest the indicator and it goes weak. This reaction is interpreted as a weakness in the digestive process in the stomach that needs attention. Such a reaction is actually very common in persons over forty, and the older the person the more common it is.[7,8]

It would be rare indeed if during an office visit with me therapy localization was not used. Here are some of the areas of the body that would commonly be therapy localized: A number of places on the head: the back of the head, the slope going up from the back of the head, the top of the head, the area above the forehead, the forehead itself, the sides of the head above the ears, the ears themselves, the eyes, the sinuses, the teeth, and the TMJ (temporomandibular joint) areas. Moving down, the cervicals; the front of the throat; the bronchial area; the lungs; the center of the sternum; the heart area; the liver area (at the bottom of the rib cage on the right side); the digestion (center just below the rib cage); the small intestines; the ascending, transverse, and descending areas of the colon; areas in the lower abdomen (these correlate with hormonal issues); along the spine; and the kidneys and adrenals in the lower back.

These and even others that I've not mentioned here are commonly tested. These points or areas of the body are usually referred to as *reflex points*. The term seems to have originated with Dr. Versendaal who referred to his work as the analysis of reflex points. I'll make use of the term from now on even though from my experience, *reflex points* seem to be more *areas on the body* rather than points. They're often directly over the organs themselves that they represent. They're also sometimes just areas of the body that through experience it has been determined what they represent and have been found to be important to test.[9] I believe there is a strong correlation between what are called reflex points and the acupuncture/meridian system.

## Turning Reflex Points On and Off

Consider a reflex point on the front of the body that tests weak. If we rub down on the point (area) it will then test strong. It's as if we turned off the reflex indication. If we then rub up, it will test weak again; we've turned it back on. By "rubbing down" or "rubbing up" I mean just taking your hand and making a motion like you were brushing away an insect. Turning reflexes on and off will have significant applications. I said above: "a reflex point on the front of the body." If we had used a reflex point on the back of the body, things would be reversed; rubbing up would turn it off and rubbing down would turn it on. Almost all of the reflex points tested are on the front of the body.

## Scoring (sometimes called Pulsing)

I don't know who deserves the credit for discovering this. To me it's second only to therapy localization in great discoveries. Here's an example of what scoring means: Let's say you find the liver reflex weak (the indicator goes weak when therapy localizing the liver area). While still therapy localizing the liver area, *I ask*: "Is the score a zero?" And test the indicator. Let's say the indicator tests strong. A few seconds ago the indicator went weak when you therapy localized the liver. Now my hand is still on the same liver area, but now I'm *asking* for different information. I'm asking about a score. The indicator (the arm) is now strong which is interpreted as the score is not a zero. If you stop and think about what I just said, this should be of great interest. I asked a question and got an answer in the form of a change in the muscle response! We'll discuss this amazing phenomenon at greater length below. But going on with the example, I then ask: "Is the score a one?" Again I test the arm and it tests strong. The score is not a one. Let's say you work your way up to asking: "Is the score a six?" and the arm drops. You can then ask if the score is a seven or any other number and the arm will test strong. It will only go down when you ask about six! So we interpret this as the score is a six! Every reflex point has a score at the moment and an optimal score, the ideal score for the reflex. The optimal score for the liver seems to be ten.

There are many questions suggested here. Who was I addressing these questions to? How do I know what the optimal scores are? How do I raise suboptimal scores? We will address these questions presently.

Since we can score any weakness found anywhere on the body at any time, we have a simple way of evaluating the effectiveness of whatever therapy is being used to raise the score! That is, we have a baseline score that later can be used to determine the value of what we're doing to try and get that score to its optimal value.[10]

I mentioned that the body has a natural score for each reflex point. For most but not all reflex points the natural scores seem mostly to be ten. The scores are always between zero to some positive value; I've never encountered a negative score; in fact I've never encountered a zero. The largest natural score I've found is associated with a person's hair which seems always to be in the range from zero to about thirty-five. Actually I've never come across a hair score as low as one or even two, but I often find the low scores of four, five or six. We find optimal hair values to be slightly different for each person, ranging from between twenty-five and thirty-five. Every male with a severe male-pattern baldness that I've tested had a hair score somewhere near five! Every child I've tested had an optimal score. I've never found a woman with a really low score, but many are not optimal.

Can a hair score be raised? From our experience, yes! At the moment I don't know how to get every hair score to its optimal value but we can raise a low score significantly. Here is an area of research with exciting possibilities.

How we find optimal scores will be discussed later.

## A Somewhat Different Application

Here's another different area of application. Dr. Anderson liked to demonstrate this in his classes.

For this demonstration we need a person wearing something that has *pants pockets*. The subject lies down and the psoas muscle is tested; let's say it's strong. The psoas muscle is a muscle that connects the upper part of the leg to the lower spine.[11] Now the subject is asked to take a short walk for about a minute *with hands in the pockets*. After this the psoas is retested and it will test weak. Now another short walk but this time the hands are not in the pockets but are now swinging naturally. After this the psoas will return to testing strong.

The lesson: Walking in what the body considers an unnatural way is not good. In particular, don't walk with your hands in your pockets! If you walk for some distance holding bundles of say of groceries this would give the same negative effect, it would be a good idea in this case after you put the bundles down to take a short walk with a natural movement of the arms to "reset" yourself. A corollary of this is bicycling is not a natural motion. Am I saying that bicycling is not a good exercise? Not necessarily; it's not a natural motion, but perhaps the aerobic benefits outweigh the downside. Also, walking on a treadmill holding onto the front bar is not completely desirable.

Walking properly is a very good exercise. Dr. Anderson called walking *"nature's chiropractic adjustment."*

# Endnotes

1. See Appendix A for some further remarks about sugar.

2. See the Appendix B on Aspartame to get some idea as to why the body might be rejecting NutriSweet.

3. See Appendix C on gluten.

4. To learn more about Nambudripad's work, contact NAET Seminars, 6714 Beach blvd., Buena Park, CA 90621

5. One of my teachers actually does suggest taking off the plastic top on any bottle being tested. I never found this to be necessary.

6. Just below the zyphoid process.

7. Antacids are the opposite of what the vast majority of persons with weak stomach digestion need. The widespread use of antacids is in my opinion the making of a widespread health disaster.

8. A few minutes ago I was taking a short break from writing and I was just outside the door near the entrance to our office. A young woman came up and asked if I spoke Spanish. I told her I was attempting to learn but I was far from fluent at this time. She asked what I did and after a short explanation she mentioned something about a severe digestive problem. I asked her to step into the waiting room and asked if I could give her a demonstration. I asked her to hold out her arm and I therapy localized the stomach reflex and it tested strong! I was very surprised, just about everyone with digestive problems will test weak on this reflex. After a little more conversation it became clear that it was her husband with the stomach problem!! Her English and my Spanish didn't intersect too well but the body's wisdom understood.

9. When the medical establishment through their testing procedures finds a problem say with a person's liver, there will be pathology, the problem will have already developed to some degree of severity. It's my opinion that the information we get from muscle-response testing can indicate weaknesses and developing problems that can be detected much before they would reach a state of some seriousness. I believe what we have with the technology I'm describing implies important new methods of disease prevention.

10. Treatment is one of the words that only licensed medical doctors are allowed by law to use. As far as I know, it's not yet against the law to improve scores or to strengthen weaknesses.

11. If Dr. Anderson asked a student to identify the psoa muscle he would expect an answer like: It's the muscle that connects the lesser trocantor of the femur at L3, L4 and L5.

# Section 5: Raising Reflex Scores

Let's say I've found a reflex point with a non-optimal score; suppose it's the liver and its score is 6. How can the score be raised? Here's what I used to do. I would take a bottle of a nutritional supplement found useful for the liver and have the person hold it near their body as we redo the scoring. It might now score at say a 9. I would say: "Great, take the supplement." Although I would consider this still a very interesting demonstration, I now have a much better way of finding what the body really needs to raise a low score and thereby become healthier.

Scoring is not part of Applied Kinesiology, but testing supplements to see if the weakness found in a muscle-response test is strengthened by it *is* part of Applied Kinesiology. But in Applied Kinesiology protocols, as I already mentioned above, it is required when testing a supplement that the supplement be *actually tasted*. It is not part of Applied Kinesiology to just hold a bottle during the test. In fact, AK rejects this kind of testing. Here's one issue where I'm parting ways with Applied Kinesiology. I find that just holding bottle of a correct supplement (there may be many different supplements that would be useful) gives a clear response from the test. If you recall the demonstration with sugar, you may wonder if we can also take this further making this even more difficult to believe by just imagining the supplement. The answer is that under certain circumstances we can, but I won't go into this at this time.

I said above that seeing if a particular supplement will raise a suboptimal score on an organ is what we used to do. At this time in our development when encountering a suboptimal score we do much more as well. I'll go into this a little more later on. I should add that this material is so new and things are developing so rapidly that the protocols we use do undergo modifications regularly. When we replace something we used to do, it's rarely a drastic change and it never invalidates what we used to do; it only makes the protocols more effective and testing situations seem to make more sense.

## Is this good for you?

With the demonstrations of sugar, NutriSweet, and the cola drinks, we saw that it's easy to test to see if the body has an *aversion* to a food, a drink, a supplement, or whatever. Can one also ask if "the body" *likes* a food, a drink, a supplement, or whatever? Yes, this is also possible! Unfortunately there is a difference between what a person likes and what the person's "body" likes.[1] One can also ask *to what degree* the item is good or bad for a particular person!

**Demonstration 7**: Suppose I want to test a nutritional supplement on a subject. He or she is asked to hold the supplement[2] while I point to the center of the slope of the subject's nose and ask: "Is this good for you?" Let's say when I do this the indicator goes weak. This may be confusing but when pointing to the nose and asking about a supplement, I now interpret a weakening as a "yes, the supplement is good for the person." The person being tested may have absolutely no idea what the supplement is or what it's supposed to be good for and this doesn't make any difference to the test. It also doesn't make any difference what I know or think about the supplement. If the indicator had stayed strong when I pointed to the nose and asked if it was good for the subject, I would interpret this as "No, it should not be taken."

Now, let's say I got a response that means it's good for the person being tested. I could then ask: "Is this really *needed*?" Not only is it good but is it needed! Again while pointing to the nose a weak response is a yes! And a strong response is a no!

Alternatively, *without pointing to the nose*, while the subject is holding the supplement to be tested, I could also have said: "Is this supplement *positive*?" Meaning, "Is it good for the person?" Here a strong response is interpreted as "Yes, it's positive. It is good for the person" A weakening of the indicator would have meant it was negative, meaning it's not good for the person. I could also at the start have asked: "Is this supplement *negative*?" I would have gotten the same information. I usually ask both questions as a redundant check on the information received.

Let's assume we're not using the "question-point" (center of the nose) and the supplement has tested positive. I can then go further and ask: "How positive is it?" "Is it between zero and ten?" If the indicator goes weak, I interpret this as: "Yes, it is between zero and ten." I would then test the numbers between zero and ten and only one value will weaken the indicator. Let's say it was seven. I would then know the item was positive and had a value of seven. So what does a +7 mean? Hold on and it should clear up. If the indicator stayed strong for values between zero and ten, I would ask about values between ten and one hundred; then between one hundred and one thousand; then between one thousand and ten thousand; and so forth. There is nothing sacred about these ranges, they're just what I use. In my experience, it often goes into the billions before the indicator weakens. I know some of you are thinking that *any* arm would weaken by the time we got into the billions! Actually, I test from 0-10, 10-100, 100-1000, 1000-10,000, 10,000-100,000, 100,000-1,000,000, 1,000,000-100,000,000, one hundred million to one billion, one billion to 100 billion, etc.

So there really isn't too much arm-pushing. When I find the right range we can then converge in to the correct value. When we get into the large number ranges, a number like 10 million is close enough and we wouldn't go further, even though the correct value may be something like 9,372,421. I also know the arm is not weakening from fatigue because as we continue the session it's again strong.

The same procedure is used to find how negative a substance is for a particular person, if of course it indicated to be negative.

One woman brought in an EPA/DHA fish oil supplement and asked if it was good for her. We found it was positive with a value of 50 million. I then tested another brand that I carry and mine tested about 60 million. I interpret this as her body really likes fish oil supplements, and mine was just a little better but maybe not significantly better.

A fellow was interested in a meal-replacement powder that I carry in the office. I believe this product is very valuable for most persons, but for him it tested only at positive three! The body was saying "It's OK but nothing to get excited about." I suggested he find something else.

At the moment these numeric values have meaning for me only in the role of comparisons. The higher the positive value the more the body seems to value the item. The same supplement can of course give different results for different persons.

What I seem to be finding is that scores in the millions and billions indicate supplements the body really needs.

Can one test persons instead of supplements? We all know that certain person's seem to drain your energy. Can the body measure this? Can one hold a photo of a person and test? How about books? Can one test to see what the body thinks of a book? What exactly can be tested besides food and food supplements? I'll leave these as open questions.[3]

## The pull-away test

Here is another test procedure to determine if a supplement is needed. I use this test usually as a double check with just about every person I'm working with to determine if a supplement, homeopathic remedy or herbal formula is needed. Suppose there's a supplement I want to test. I hold the bottle near the person and test an indicator, if it goes weak the supplement is not for the person. If the indicator stays strong I then pull the supplement away from the body simultaneously testing an indicator. If the indicator goes weak as I pull it away from the body, I interpret this response as: "the supplement is really needed!" It's not only good for the person, but the body has a strong need for it. It's as if the body is saying: "Don't take it away, I need it!"

# Endnotes

1. I believe when the body likes or needs something, it's because of a health issue that needs improvement.

2. Holding the supplement can mean holding an actual tablet, capsule or whatever. It can mean holding a bottle of the substance even if the bottle is in its packaging. It can even mean more than this, but let's not go there.

3. The book Power versus Force by David Hawkins, Hay House, 1995, addresses some of these questions.

# Section 6: Asking Questions

*"The individual human mind is like a computer terminal connected to a giant database. The database is human consciousness itself, of which our own cognizance is merely an individual expression, but with its roots in the common consciousness of all mankind. This database is the realm of genius; because to be human is to participate in the database, everyone, by virtue of his birth, has access to genius. The unlimited information contained in the database has now been shown to be readily available to anyone in a few seconds, at any time and in any place. This is indeed an astonishing discovery, bearing the power to change lives, both individually and collectively, to a degree never yet anticipated."*

*Dr. David Hawkins from Power vs Force.*

In the seminars of the Walker's, on their *Neuro-Emotional Technique*® (NET), it's emphasized that in doing a muscle-response test, one is never asking a question. Rather statements are made by the practitioner or the subject and if a statement results in the indicator going weak, the subject is said to be "not congruent" with the statement. If the muscle stays strong, the subject is "congruent" with the statement. Not being congruent with a statement can be thought of as the statement triggering a response indicating the statement has a "charge" or is "hot" probably only in the subconscious and this needs to be "corrected." There is not necessarily a correlation with what the subject consciously believes and congruence. "I'm OK with my current job," and the arm drops. "I'm OK with giving up sugar," and the arm drops. "I'm perfectly happy with my life as it is," and the arm drops. The arm may also drop when saying: "I really want to be well," "I really want to give up smoking," or "I really want to lose weight." I'll be getting into this topic in some detail below; for now I just wanted to say a few words about asking questions with muscle-response testing.

Asking questions is also not part of Applied Kinesiology although testing a muscle to determine if an organ may need attention seems to me to imply a non-verbal question.

*Some of us, on the other hand, as you obviously have already gathered, have no problem with asking questions.*

You'll recall that when doing a "battery test" I pointed to the area between the eyes and ask, usually silently: "May I communicate with this person?" This is asking a question, but we can take this further – much further!

*When pointing to the battery tester point we can ask many other questions as well and not just about whether or not we're communicating!!*

In this case, *a strong response is interpreted as a NO, and a weak response is a YES.* We don't know the limitations on this facility at the moment, but this is a major and in fact an indispensable tool that I use a great deal. This is one of the many discoveries made by Dr. Melnicke. Actually, according to him the exact place to point for asking questions is at the center of the slope of the nose, a little below the battery tester point. From my experience, the body seems to accept the battery tester point as being close enough.

# Section 7: More on Raising Reflex Scores

**Will this supplement help?**

We've already discussed this above, but let's take another look. I find an organ in need of help. What help can I offer? There are many possibilites: Certain nutritional supplements may help; dietary improvements may help; herbal formulas may help; homeopathy may help; detoxification may help; chiropractic may help; exercise may help; stress reduction may help; emotional work may help; acupuncture may help; it may even be the case that drugs may help (these of course would be prescribed only by a licensed medical doctor).

When an organ is indicating a dysfunction, by which I usually mean that therapy localizing the organ gives a weakness in the indicator, as I said earlier I do not now in my current stage of development just test to see if a supplement will help strengthen the muscle-response, although in the early days I would do this. Now I use a more complex procedure. One should not, therefore, read too much into the following example.

Let's say the liver therapy localizes weak. I then have the subject hold a bottle of tablets of let's say it's an herbal formula intended to cleanse and strengthen the liver and I retest and now the therapy localization gives a strong response. I interpret this as the herbal formula will help the liver. There are many other possibilities I could have used in place of the herbal formula. If I had tested several of the possibilities, I might want to know which of these the body prefers. This also can be done and I'll show you how shortly.

**Causal Chains**

In order to help the liver, the digestion may be causing problems for the liver and it needs to be strengthened first. This may be the only reason why the liver is in need of help. On the other hand, the digestive weakness may be caused by a leaky gut which may in turn be caused by excess stress, and the excess stress may be caused by any number of other factors. Of course, I'm using the liver as an example and any other organ would require the same kind of considerations.

## More on Correcting Weaknesses

A reflex point that therapy localizes weak is of course indicating a weakness of whatever part of the body correlates to the reflex. A reflex point with a suboptimal score would also indicate a weakness in the corresponding organ, the lower the score the more the organ is in need of help. But *a reflex point with a low score does not always therapy localize as a weakness.* Why should this be? The most common reason is that the body's wisdom is telling us that something else needs to be attended to first and it may be counterproductive to go out of order. A very common example of this is that the liver on a person may have a low score but will not therapy localize as a weakness, but the gallbladder *will* therapy localize as a weakness. After erasing the gallbladder reflex then the liver will show the weakness. The body's wisdom is telling us that we should not be helping the liver if the gallbladder is not helped first. This implies that all weaknesses might be prioritized by the body's innate intelligence and this is indeed possible.

## Priority and the K27 Points

K27 are two very important acupuncture points located bilaterally just below the collar bone near the edge of the sternum. Let's say I had scanned all reflex points on a client and found a number of weaknesses. If I then asked the client to put a thumb and pointer finger on the K27 points then while the client is holding these points, only one of the weaknesses would still test weak and all the rest will now test strong. The one weakness will indicate the reflex that is most in need of attention, the first priority.

You may recall the concept of erasing a reflex introduced above. Here's a good example of using this. Suppose we've found the most important reflex using the K27 points and we determined that other reflexes need to be dealt with in order to properly help the most important reflex.[1] If we then erase this most important reflex, the body will then temporarily consider this weakness fixed and will then show you the next reflex that needs attention. This will also be the only reflex you will find in this situation.[2]

Suppose one erased a reflex and forgot to get the score. You can restore what you erased returning the reflex to its original condition my just rubbing up on the reflex. You can then test for the score. So rubbing down on a reflex turns it off and rubbing up turns it back on.[3]

We have entered on a topic that gets rather involved. Working to improve the score of a reflex, say the most important reflex, usually improves other reflexes as well. Also improving the score of any reflex often requires other reflexes also be addressed. It's also important to know when you've addressed enough issues for a particular office visit. Finding the answer to this question is possible also. It's almost always not productive to try and address too much all at once on one office visit. I'll have more to say on this in Section 11.

## Endnotes

1. Remember this is only a guided tour and I can't do justice to every hypothesized situation.

2. Here is an area where the protocol has been significantly improved. Explaining this will also have to wait for another time.

3. I'm thinking only of reflexes on the front of the body.

# Section 8: What's It's Natural Score?

**Giving Temporary Energy**

Chi Gong is a major therapeutic tool used by the Taoist physician. It can briefly be described as ancient Chinese exercises combining meditation and slow movements. Tai Chi is a well-known form of Chi Gong. The purpose of Chi Gong is essentially to amplify and facilitate the flow of the Qi energy in the body. A fundamental positioning of the body in Chi Gong involving no movement at all is called the *Wu Chi* position. The part of this position relevant here is that the person's arms are held stationary as if they were hugging an imaginary tree. This position together with proper breathing is believed to maximize (at least temporarily) the flow of Qi in the body.

The point of introducing this here is: In this position there is a strong flow of Qi between the hands! We can make use of this to energize areas of the body!

**Demonstration 8: Finding Natural Scores**

Let's say we test the score of a person's hair. This is done by lightly pinching a small amount of the person's hair and then doing the scoring procedure. Let's say the score comes out to four.[1] I then put my hands near but not touching on each side of his head in the area above each ear. My arms and hands are in a position similar to how they would be in the Wu Chi position. Holding my hands still I then breathe deeply from the lower diaphragm for about twenty seconds. When I retest the hair I'll get what I believe to be the natural score, i.e., the perfect score for that person; unfortunately it is only an indication of what the score should be; it is not a procedure for actually raising this score. A perfect hair score is usually in the range from 25 to 35.

*This technique can be used to find the natural score of any reflex.*

I should think there would be considerable interest in raising the score of hair and certainly not only with men. I said I know how to raise a low score on a person's hair but can I raise a hair score to its optimal score? I haven't been able to yet, but I'm hopeful. What would happen if we could raise the score of a person with male-pattern baldness to its optimal value through health improvement? It's not only an intriguing hypothetical question but it's a research problem waiting to be worked on.

# Endnotes

1. I tested the score of a fellow two days ago that had a severe case of the common male baldness pattern. His hair tested 4 and his natural score was 25!

# Section 9: My Tool Kit

My whole practice can be considered exclusively focused on raising scores of reflexes.

So how do I raise scores? My "tool kit" consists of:

- Nutritional supplements, almost entirely *whole-food* nutritional supplements;
- Dietary advice;
- Herbal formulas;
- Homeopathic remedies;
- Advice on detoxification;
- Advice on exercising;
- Advice on stress-management; and
- Emotional clearings, which will be discussed in some detail below.

The whole-food supplements I use are almost exclusively from *Standard Process®*, a company in Wisconsin founded by Dr. Royal Lee about seventy-five years ago. In my opinion, Dr. Lee was the greatest scientist in the field of nutrition of all time. He's no longer with us, but his company is still thriving, now under the direction of some of his family members who continue to make a large number of different whole-food nutritional supplements, most of which were designed by Dr. Lee. Although there are some whole-food supplements available from other companies that I also use, Standard Process is unique in many of their formulas and in the large number of different formulas made available. From my experience, for any physical problem I may find with a client, there will always be some Standard Process products that can help. My hope is that some day there will be many more companies that follow Dr. Lee's lead and market similar whole-food supplements. I'm far from the only practitioner with such a high regard for Dr. Lee and his work, almost every Applied Kinesiologist and almost every one doing work with muscle-response testing that I know uses Standard Process products.[1]

45

## Which Do You Like Better?

Recall the "Pull-Away Test"? I hold a supplement near a person and the indicator is strong, then as I pull the supplement away from the person's body the indicator goes weak. My interpretation of the arm going weak in this situation is that the body is telling me: "Please don't take it away I need it!"

Here's a variation of this test that is not only a remarkable demonstration of the value of Standard Process products, but it's also one of my most useful tools.

**Demonstration 9**: I get a bottle of a top quality vitamin E supplement. It contains 400 units of alpha tocopherol together with the synergistic mineral selenium. I also get a bottle of Standard Process' Cataplex® E which is a whole-food supplement that can be considered Dr. Lee's vitamin E supplement. It contains only *5 units* of what's called vitamin E as opposed to the 400 units in the other supplement. It also contains some naturally occurring selenium. Here's the test: The subject holds the Cataplex E and the indicator tests strong. I then bring the bottle of the 400 unit supplement near the subject's body and slowly move it away simultaneously testing an indicator and the indicator stays strong. Now I reverse things; the subject holds the 400 unit supplement and as I move the Cataplex E away from the subject's body and the indicator goes weak! The body seems to be saying: "Please don't take the Cataplex E away, I like it better!"

## Herbal Formulas

Then there are herbal formulas. In my office I have an extensive variety of individual herbal extracts and herbal formulas. The individual herbal extracts are used almost exclusively to make individualized formulas. Classical Chinese medicine also seldom uses herbs individually. Diet therapy and herbal therapy are closely related, in fact, I consider all the herbs I use special foods. In classical Chinese medicine, the two primary tools used by the physician are diet and herbs and they also don't distinguish between the two very much. Medicinal herbs are, for example, used regularly in Taoist cooking.[2] Dr. Stephen Chang, a famous Taoist physician and one of my teachers, calls herbs "super foods."

There is at this time in our country a growing interest in medicinal herbs, but unfortunately not by our mainstream health care system. I predict we will see this interest continue to grow,[3] paralleling that which occurred with acupuncture. Perhaps it is not impossible that some day we will see a shift to the use of herbal medicine by our health care system so dominated at present by the use of drugs.

Some of my favorite formulas (mostly liquid extracts) are:

- Eleuthro root, Oat milky seed, Schesandra fruit, Gotu Kola aerial parts, Rhodiola root, and American Ginseng root (mainly an adrenal tonic)[4]
- Hawthorn fruit, leaf, and flower; Linden flower, Night-Blooming Cereus stem, Ginkgo leaf, Prickley Ash bark, and Bugleweed aerial parts (a heart tonic)[4]
- Saw Palmetto fruit, White Sage aerial parts, Collinsonia whole plant, and Stinging Nettles root (a prostate formula)[4]
- St. John's Wort flowers, Lomatum root, Hyssop aerial parts, Lemon Balm aerial parts, and Isadis root (an antiviral formula)[4]
- Dandelion root, Gentian root, Artichoke leaf, Orange peel, Angelica root, and Peppermint aerial parts (a digestive aid)[1]
- Dandelion root, Watercress aerial parts, Blessed Thistle aerial parts, Milk Thistle seed, Turmeric rhizome, and Oregon Grape root (a liver tonic)[4]

There are actually a great many more formulas that should be on this list.

**Nutrition and Diet**

> *"If you always do what you've always done, You'll always get what you've always got."*
>
> *Annonymous*

In my opinion, the *Standard American Diet* is a major cause, and perhaps *the* major cause of most of the health problems in this country. It certainly isn't the only cause, but I don't consider any other factor more important, although pollution is a possibility. Improving the diet is a powerful therapeutic tool and almost every client I see does need to make major dietary improvements. I use the word "need" in the sense that no substantial, long term health improvements are possible while continuing on a poor diet. From my experience there are very few persons that can make many substantial dietary changes all at once. The process toward a healthful diet in almost all cases can only be sustained through a carefully and individually designed plan, and implemented at a comfortable pace.

There is of course no diet right for everyone, but here are some suggestions that would apply to just about everyone, and if followed rigorously would result in major improvements in a person's diet together with the resulting health improvements. The suggestions are easily stated, but implementing them would take much commitment.

### *Get sugar, trans-fats and white flour out of your life.*

About 10% of all the calories in the standard American diet are from sugar, about 30% is from white flour products, and trans-fats are in just about every processed food item. It's not too difficult to believe the percentage on the white flour products if you consider the breads, bagels, pasta, donuts, cakes, pretzels, cookies, and pizza. The sugar percentage can be stated in another way: The average American eats his or her weight each year in sugar! Soft drinks and sugary desserts are major sources. I think the main reason why the low-carbohydrate diets do "work" is because they do cut out the sugar and white flour products.

But things are never so simple. Which of the following two possibilities is better: A poor diet and a strong digestive system or an excellent diet with a weak digestive system? I think it's the poor diet with the strong digestion. If a person has weak digestion and a poor diet, then making improvements in the diet while ignoring the digestive problem is not reasonable. Improving the digestive system might not be so easy; it might require strengthening the liver function, or it might require reducing negative stress in the person's life, or it might require eliminating food intolerances, or it might require any number of other possibilities. This raises another question: When a person needs to improve his or her health, what needs to be done first? Certainly any improvement anywhere is always positive, but clearly the most pressing weaknesses should be attended to first. Fortunately the body's intelligence can help us sort all this out. More on these thoughts below.

## Homeopathy

Homeopathy is another major tool I use on just about every person I see in my practice. Homeopathy has the potential to help with *any* health problem, including those considered to be in the mental/emotional domain.

Homeopathy is a somewhat ambiguous term that does not denote a unique system of healing. Roughly there are two kinds of homeopathy, one referred to as "classical" homeopathy and is based on the teachings of the founder of Homeopathy, Samuel Hahnemann (1754 -1843), as set forth in his *Organon of Medicine*. The main distinguishing feature of classical homeopathy is the use of a single remedy at a time chosen on the symptom picture of the client.

Then there are those that use mixtures of homeopathic remedies. The classical homeopath does not consider this kind of practice to be "homeopathy" since it cannot be justified from the Organon. I've had training in both schools and I'm convinced there is merit in each camp, but at the moment I'm mostly in the classical camp and I do use only a single remedy at a time. Then again I'm in neither camp since I use muscle-response testing with homeopathy as well as everything else. I once told one of my teachers (of Homeopathy) that I believed the greatest discovery in homeopathy since the time of Hahnemann might be the application of muscle-response testing to finding the correct homeopathic remedy. He didn't get very excited by what I said, but I'm even more convinced this is true than I was then.

I mentioned homeopathic remedies and I should say a few words about this. Homeopathic remedies are commonly sold in the form of tubes containing small pills. Although I use homeopathic remedies only in liquid form, I believe it doesn't make much difference which form one uses. Homeopathic remedies are sometimes confused with herbal remedies, but there is no similarity. The therapeutic value in herbs are mostly in its phytochemicals and I believe herbs work mostly in the physical domain. Homeopathy, on the other hand works *only* in a non-physical, "energetic" domain. If one had any homeopathic remedy tested in any chemical laboratory, there would be nothing found but water and alcohol in the liquid remedies and only a kind of sugar in the small pills. But homeopathic remedies contain powerful vibrational energies that can be of enormous value in the hands of an experienced homeopath. Homeopathy is extremely safe, being virtually free of negative side effects.

This certainly needs more discussion if you're new to this:

Homeopathy is based on what is called the *law of similars*, which (very briefly) is that a substance capable of producing certain symptoms in a healthy person, is capable, in very small doses, of curing a sick person who displays similar symptoms. Here are a few very simple examples:

(1) You have coffee too close to bedtime and you can't sleep. You take a homeopathic remedy made from coffee.
(2) You have a running nose caused by a cold. You take a homeopathic remedy made from onion!

The belief in a self-healing power within the human body is of prime importance in homeopathy, and the homeopath's interpretation of symptoms is very different from that of mainstream medicine where *symptoms are the problem* and are treated. If you have a fever, it is to be lowered. If you have diarrhea, it is to be stopped. If you have a pain it is to be covered over. Since the homeopath believes that the vital force always strives for cure, for harmony and balance in the functioning of the body, to the homeopath the *symptoms of disease are the signs of the curative process*. The states of what we call disease are actually indications of the modes the body uses to try and restore itself to health. To the homeopath the symptoms indicate the route taken by the body in combating an imbalance and are the best guides to homeopathic treatment. The homeopath tries to find the homeopathic remedy made from a substance that would cause a similar symptom picture if given in non-homeopathic doses. The aim of the homeopathic physician then is to stimulate the body's own defense mechanism, and the curative remedy is the one which supports the body's inherent but at time insufficient healing effort. *Homeopathy then is systematic support to the self-healing efforts of the body.*

I'm sure I've raised more questions than I've answered on homeopathy; fortunately there are many good books available. For example, you might want to read *Homeopathy: Medicine for the Modern Man*, or better still, although more scholarly: *The Science of Homeopathy*, both by George Vithoulkas, for a more complete understanding of the topic.

_Serafino Amoroso_

# Endnotes

1. I have no financial ties to this or any other company.

2. They're actually used in all the cuisines of the world (parsley, thyme, garlic, etc.).

3. I also expect a lot of opposition from opposing commercial interests.

4. Designed by David Winston

# Section 10: The Mental/Emotional Domain

For the mental- emotional domain we also have the work of Dr. Scott Walker who along with his wife Dr. Debbie Walker DC and Dr. Daniel Monti MD offer seminars throughout the country on what they call *NET®* (*Neuro-Emotional Technique*).[1,2] I highly recommend any health care professional consider taking at least their Basic NET Seminar.

NET is almost exclusively the work of Dr. Scott Walker which he introduced in the late 1980's and that he and others continue to develop. Papers are now being published on aspects of this work in the mainstream research literature. Although Dr. Walker is clearly the driving force behind this work, he has borrowed much, especially from traditional Chinese medicine.

## What Are Neuro-Emotional Clearings?

As we go through life we all experience with varying degrees of intensity much emotional trauma. If I asked you to recall such an event from your past, or even the present, you quite likely would be able to recall not only the event but would be able as well to actually re-experience exactly how you felt at the time it happened. Many of these events are *unresolved emotional trauma*. What would make them *unresolved* for us would be a weakening of an indicator as the event is mentally recalled. We who use this technique believe that unresolved emotional trauma, even though it mostly remains in the subconscious, can still have an adverse effect on your health in at least the following way. Each of the unresolved emotional trauma has what we can call a *pattern* and when something happens in your daily life that resonates with this pattern, i.e., reminds the body (the subconscious) of the original event, the current event will have a much more exaggerated, negative physiological effect than it should have.

Dr. Walker has developed a technique to resolve the emotional trauma by removing the "emotional charges" from these subconscious memories. The manifestation of the charge being removed is that an indicator will no longer weaken as it did before the clearing. I feel this procedure should be routinely used as part of any health improvement plan, and I very much hope that this technique will soon become part of the tool-kit of every health care provider. It would be especially appropriate for a therapist and perhaps every spiritual counselor also (priest, minister).

It should be made clear that what I'll be discussing here has nothing to do with mental illness, nor even with psychological problems.

What I'm going to describe now should not be considered Dr. Walker's "official" NET. The Walkers have worked very hard to develop their Neuro Emotional Technique and naturally want to exercise quality control over their product. What I'm going to describe can only give a rough indication of their work. Although you might want to look at their website (www.netbodymind.com) for more official information, there is no substitute for taking their seminar. But I hope what I'm presenting here is close enough to give you a feel for the procedure and to spark your interest. Again, it is not my intention to be teaching you how to perform clearings, official or otherwise.

So far it would seem that we've been concerned exclusively with the physical body, with the digestion, the liver, the adrenals, the hair, and so forth. One might say that now we will be discussing part of the non-physical domain of the body. This is in a sense correct, but it should be understood that the non-physical (which includes the mental/emotional domain) is so intertwined with the physical that it is wrong to think they can be separated. You can't improve the physical body without the side effect of helping the mental/emotional body, and you can't help the mental/emotional without the side effect of improving the physical body as well.

**Demonstration 10:** Test an indicator muscle on a test subject (let's say her name is Mary) and let's say you find it strong. Now have the test subject say "My name is Mary" and the indicator will remain strong. Now have Mary say "My name is Jane" or Harriet or any other name. The indicator will go weak! [3]

This is a normal reaction. I just mention this as an illustration of what happens when persons make a statement to which they are "incongruent."

Remember I'm just giving you a tour and stopping at some highlights. There will be many implications that may occur to you as we go along. It's also likely that many of these implications will not as yet have been explored.

In general again, without getting into the subject too deeply, let's consider Scott Walker's OK-statements. For example, the subject makes a statement like: "I'm OK with my present weight," or "I'm OK if I never lose weight." Any person should test strong on these OK statements no matter how much or how little the person wants to or needs to lose weight. In fact, everyone should test strong on *every* positively phrased OK-statement no matter what it is. Why is this so? Such statements do not indicate preference; for example, you should still test strong on the OK statements above even if you are very unhappy with your present weight. Weakening on an OK-statement seems to indicate an over-concern with the issue, and it's perhaps the over-concern that needs to be corrected. Dr. Walker gives an interesting example of an Olympic runner that improved his running times when cleared for a weakening on the statement: "I'm OK if I *lose* a match." One might also weaken on the statement: "I'm OK if I *win* a match." There are an almost unlimited number of OK-statements that can be tested.

**Demonstration 11: Recalling Emotional Trauma**

Have the subject think of some emotionally traumatic event that happened sometime in the person's life; it doesn't matter how distant in the past. The more severe the event the more likely the indicator will go weak. If the indicator does go weak as the subject recalls the event, this is the situation we described above by saying there's a "charge" on the memory of the event; or the event has not been "resolved." Let's now take a look at my unofficial description of the technique for taking the charge off the memory of such events.

Having the person choose a traumatic event is perhaps the most direct way of finding what Dr. Walker calls a *neuro-emotional complex* or an *NEC*; there are several other ways as well. NEC's can be considered events that have happened in the person's past that have never been properly "resolved." When the person is reminded of such an event, as I've already mentioned, he or she can recall not only the event but can re-experience the emotions that were felt at the time - there may be a complex of emotions involved with the event and not just one.

When Scott Walker first introduced means of "clearing" NEC's, his technique was quite physical, using what he considered chiropractic adjustments. I would consider those techniques closer to the topic of acupuncture, but in any case he later introduced an alterative method that was far less physical. This new technique also borrowed from traditional Chinese medicine.

From the beginning, Dr. Walker based his work on the Taoist belief that there is a set of emotions associated with each segment of the meridian system. Experiencing these emotions has a direct effect on the energy flow in the corresponding meridian segment. We have just a hint in our culture of the correctness of this belief. We all know that extreme excitement can affect the heart, also extreme fear can affect the bladder (can this not make persons wet their pants?), and hopelessness or worry can affect the digestion. Traditional Chinese medicine over the millennia have worked out this association in great detail going far beyond these meager examples, and this knowledge forms an essential part of this emotional clearing technique.

I said there are several other ways of finding NEC's; here's another: Suppose while testing a person's reflex points you find say a weakness in the liver. It could have been any other reflex point as well but let's say the liver. So when you place your hand near the liver area the indicator goes weak. Now you ask the subject to place a hand flat on their forehead. When you then retest the liver the indicator is now strong. This is interpreted as an NEC exists that is affecting (the energy flowing to) the liver. You could then go through the clearing process which takes an average less than ten minutes, and after this the liver score will have increased. But also if you repeat the test for an emotional component on the liver, it will now come out negative.

An important part of the last description was the subject placing a hand flat on their forehead. There are two points on the forehead, roughly one above each eye in the center of the forehead, that are associated with emotional concerns. These two points are used in every aspect of NET.

## A Typical Emotional Clearing

I'll try now to give you a general idea of what an emotional clearing is like. To describe the process with a precision that would enable you to perform one would be difficult and this is not my intention here.

Let's say we found an emotional component associated with the adrenals, that is, the adrenals tested weak, but when a hand was placed on the forehead they then tested strong. To explore the associated NEC, the practitioner first tests to see which category the event falls into. All testing is of course using muscle-response testing. There are three such categories: The issue may have something to do with *some aspect of the material world*, or it may have something to do with *an issue involving love*, or it may have something to do with *some role in life* of the person being tested. I would then test the categories by saying: "Some aspect of the material world like money, job, finances or career." If the indicator goes weak, the issue is in this category. Dr. Walker, as I mentioned earlier, emphasizes that we should not be asking questions! We should just make statements that either hit a "nerve," so to speak, or doesn't. If the indicator does not go weak on this first category, then I would make a statement relating to the second category like: "Anyone you've ever loved or anyone who's ever loved you." If this does not indicate (the arm stays strong), then I would go to the last possibility, saying: "Something about you." One of these three categories will indicate with an inhibited indicator. Let's say for the sake of our example, that the third category indicated, that is, when I said: "Something about you" the arm dropped. Then I would go on to say something like: "You have many roles in life: Your role as a mother (or as a father). If the role as mother (father) doesn't indicate, I ask about other possible roles, daughter (son), husband (wife), victim, employee, etc, etc. If I can't find a role, I take a different path. I should say here that we are trying to find hints to help the person find the event in question. Continuing, I could then "ask" about the year the event happened: "Conception to ten years old." If the body does not indicate (the indicator does not go weak), then I say: "Ten years old to twenty." Let's say I get an indication here (the arm drops). I then say: "Ten" and test the indicator; then "eleven" and test the indicator; then "twelve" etc. The indicator will go down on an age between ten and twenty, let's say eighteen. The person may at this point have a good idea what the event is that we are going after when we get to the year, but usually more information is needed. This we do by getting an emotion connected to the event. This is done though the acupuncture meridian system.

To explain this, I have to take a short detour into the Chinese wrist points which is a means of gaining access into the meridian system. From traditional Chinese medicine, there are three points on each wrist that with either shallow or deeper pressure will access different segments of the meridian system. Dr. Walker has recently added a fourth point that is as far as I know not part of classical Chinese teaching, but it seems to work as he applies it. I might say here that *pulse diagnosis* through these wrist points is the most important of all the assessment techniques used in Traditional Chinese medicine. It can be used to indicate to the experienced TCM (traditional Chinese medicine) physician *any* health-relevant issue.

Traditional Chinese medicine has long known that each segment of the meridian system has an associated set of emotions. There are charts available based on this traditional knowledge made available from Dr. Walker that show the location of the pulse points and their association with the meridian segments and the related emotions.

## Getting back now to our example:

In the context of the clearing going on in this example, when I said "eighteen," the indicator weakened. It must then be determined which pulse point will change the strength of the indicator (to strong) when saying "eighteen." If the arm still weakens when touching a wrist point, this is not the point we're looking for. The wrist point that does change the reaction of the indicator will lead via the chart to a list of emotions like anger, fear, depression, etc., and it must then be determined which emotion is associated with the issue at hand. This is done by just stating each emotion in turn from the chart and simultaneously checking the indicator. As soon as the arm drops, we have the emotion. Now the subject has another clue along with age eighteen to help in recalling the event. It is likely that some possibilities will occur to the subject. By the person just mentioning some possibilities in turn, the practitioner can determine by the reaction of the indicator if the relevant event has been found. Even when the relevant event has been found the clearing procedure can't yet begin. One has to determine first if there is an original event that has an NEC with a pattern similar to the one just determined. If there is, it's this original event that has to be found and this is the one used in the clearing process.

When we find the event that is to be cleared, and this is done in much the same way as just described, the clearing is performed as follows. The subject of the clearing is asked to do three things: Mentally go back to the original event holding (1) the emotional feeling associated with the event that indicated through the wrist point, (2) simultaneously hold the relevant wrist point and the emotional acupuncture points on the forehead, and (3) finally and simultaneously taking some deep breaths. The subject is told to do all this for a minute or so. The emotion often fades and becomes more difficult to hold and this is a reasonable time to discontinue the clearing process. After the clearing is completed, everything that weakened the person before the clearing now no longer does. For example, now saying "eighteen" keeps the indicator strong. Mentioning the emotion also now has no effect. Thinking of either the first event or the original event which previously weakened the indicator, now does not. Dr. Walker tells us that when an NEC is cleared it never needs to be cleared again, that is, it will never again indicate. From my experience he's correct.

This should give you a rough idea of what an official NET clearing is like.

There's a lot more about NET I haven't even hinted at here. One of these is the non-classical use of homeopathics. I enthusiastically recommend all of Dr. Walker's seminars where all their work is covered in a clear and useful manner.

Whenever an emotional clearing is successfully completed that originated from a weak organ (body entry), the score on the organ will increase. Just yesterday I did an emotional clearing on a woman's thymus area that had tested @10. After the clearing the score tested @ 15.

## Dreams

Dreams have long been considered an important means of communication with the subconscious, especially in what are often thought of as primitive cultures. Working with dreams is one of the latest ways of arriving at NEC's. This is a fascinating new area of research in NET.

So far there has never been a person on whom I could not find a neuro-emotional complex. This is usually an important part of raising a score on most reflex indications. I might add that practically all clients find emotional clearing to be the part of my practice they find the most interesting.

# Endnotes

1. The work of Dr. John Diamond is also more than relevant here, but I don't feel qualified to discuss his work. I would urge any health care practitioner to investigate the possibility of studying with Dr. Diamond. He holds seminars on a regular schedule and has written several books some of which are listed in the references.

2. See Appendix E

3. A controlled clinical trial along this same line was published in the Journal of Perceptual and Motor Skills, 1999, 88, 1010-1028.

# Section 11:  Constructing a Holistic Health Care Practice (Some Preliminaries)

There are different ways that health concerns can be classified. Mainstream medicine classifies health concerns by putting names on certain collections of symptoms. You have "MS," "atherosclerosis," or "hypertension," or "lupus," or whatever, and there are protocols, usually drug therapy or surgery, that are recommended for each named condition.

Another very different way is to see health issues is as the body requiring either *cleansing* (an internal detoxification), or *nourishment* (a physiological strengthening) or both. If suitably generalized I believe detoxification and nourishment do cover most health concerns. It might be argued: "What about emotional health?" I think this can be looked on as requiring a combination of different kinds of cleansing and nourishment. What I'm saying here is based on a belief that the natural state of the body is one of perfect health, and the body is self-healing with a strong tendency to move toward this state of perfect health. But to help the body requires your cooperation, which implies a lot on your part if you expect a lot.

I think it's also useful to classify health concerns into three categories, and this is the way I visualize my practice. Consider the mental picture of a triangle that is sliced horizontally into three sections: the top peak of the triangle, the middle layer, and the larger base of the triangle. In my practice I address the health concerns in the middle and base areas, but not in the top of the triangle. The top of the triangle represents acute or severe health concerns that require immediate attention, like a tooth ache or severe and debilitating back pain, or the needs associated with any of the stages of a possibly fatal illness. It's always best to find and correct the underlying causes of any health problem, but situations that fall into this top category usually require immediate attention and almost always symptom relief. Of course you can simultaneously be doing more than symptom relief, but these acute, disabling problems must be treated in the most direct manner, even if the causes are not considered.

Examples of concerns in the middle area would be a liver that is not functioning as well as it should, even though no noticeable symptoms exist, and even though medical tests may come out negative; or arteries of the heart and elsewhere in the body that are on the way to getting clogged but are not yet near a point of immediate concern; or perhaps your body is under so much stress that your adrenal glands badly need support. There are a great many more examples that I would place in the middle section of the triangle.

I'm also very much interested in the base area of the triangle. Here we find the general lifestyle issues such as diet, exercise, stress reduction, and hygiene.

**What to do first?**

Some day someone should do a definitive study of the question: "What needs to be done first for general health improvement?" I think it's an important question and I certainly don't feel comfortable trying to answer it. How about "Improve the diet first!" But then shouldn't a weak digestion be addressed before dietary improvements? Or shouldn't stress be dealt with first if it's causing the weak digestion? But then stress is so multifaceted. Perhaps a serious part of the stress is a polluted local environment, like a moldy workplace or even a moldy home. What if the person is in severe pain; should that not that be handled first even if what is done is not getting at the cause? What if a person is in need of serious dental work, or a required surgical operation? Should these not be first? What if a person just doesn't have what it takes to change a behavior that is destroying his or her health? Can anything be done in this case and if so is this not a candidate for being first?

There is another way of looking at all this that should help one not despair. I call it the "All the Holes in the Boat" principle.

Picture you're in a rowboat in the middle of a lake and the boat has many holes in its bottom but you have a coffee can that you're using to bail out the boat. You're working very hard and if the water overwhelms your efforts you're finished! Now *any* hole that you can plug up will help you survive longer. The bigger the hole you fix the better off you will be. As you plug up holes, you won't have to work so hard, you will last longer, and your life will be more pleasant. So in a sense it doesn't matter where you start as long as you don't work so slowly that you sink.

Perhaps the following is a better way to picture the situation. Visualize a large sheet of paper on which are drawn a few dozen circles of various sizes. The picture is to represent a particular person's health at a particular moment and different persons will surely have different pictures. The circles will represent the reflex areas that we test on a client. The smaller the circle the healthier the part of the body (e.g., an organ) for the client associated with the picture. A dot represents a reflex that needs no help. There will almost always be circles larger than a dot and the larger the circle the more the reflex is in need of help. So there will be spread around the paper circles of various sizes.

Now a person is not the same as a car to this extent: In a car the headlights have nothing to do with the tires, and the tires have nothing to do with the carburetor. With a person everything is interconnected. "Anything can cause anything!"

Now getting back to our picture:

If one reflex circle affects another then in our picture we draw an arrow starting at the first circle and pointing to the affected second circle. But then every circle will then have arrows leaving going to all the other circles, since anything can affect anything to some extent. Since all reflexes do not affect all others with equal intensity, we will use arrows of various thicknesses. If one reflex has a strong affect on another then the arrow will be thick. If less so, then the arrow will be thinner. If the interaction is remote, the arrow will be very thin.

It's still true that no matter what hole you plug up (i.e., make the circle smaller in this metaphor), the client will be helped, but the total picture is now more complex. Here if there's a thick arrow pointing from circle A to circle B, if we help circle A we will be helping circle B as well.

So we have a very complex picture with circles of various sizes and arrows of various thicknesses pointing all over the place. We want to help this person, so how can we proceed? What reflexes should we work on for best and quickest results?

Here is what we can do: We can ask the body's intelligence to help us. We ask: "What reflex do you suggest is the most important one to concentrate on at this moment? What associated reflexes need to be attended to in order to help the most important one?

So an answer we might get is: "Reflex X is the most important one you should concentrate on, but reflexes Y and Z (both of which have thick arrows pointing to X need to be attended to as well. And there is a thick arrow from reflex W going to reflex Z that you must attend to as well."

It's often the case that strengthening only the associated reflexes (Y, Z and W in our example above) will be sufficient to fully satisfy the main reflex X (this will change X from a large circle to a smaller one – hopefully to a dot).

Without the help from the body's intelligence (*which we can get*), much guess work would be involved that would be more or less useful.

But there are preliminaries which must come first. Most of the time I'll start with an evaluation of the autonomic nervous system. There are muscle-response tests (for example in Applied Kinesiology) that indicate how well (or how poorly) a person's physiology is responding to stress. There is also an accurate *computerized* method of testing this that I use in my practice as well.[1] Before we go on here, let's take a detour and say something about stress.

## Stress

Everyone has it, everyone talks about it, yet few really know the precise definition of stress. The word *stress* was introduced into the context of health only in the 1930's mainly by the pioneering work of the Canadian scientist, Hans Selye who was the first to make the study of stress a scientific discipline.

The term stress was borrowed from engineering: Consider a steel beam supported at both ends and with a load positioned in the center of the beam. The load is putting pressure on the beam. If the pressure is slight, there is no real affect on the beam. As the load is increased the beam may bend and if the load is increased to where the beam can no longer resist, the beam can break. It's the beam that's under stress; the load is not the stress, it's the cause of the stress, but the stress is in the beam. The load is called a *stressor*. The beam without the load is in a relaxed state and with the load it goes into a tension that is the stress.

In the context of health when we speak of stressors, we of course go well beyond a person carrying a heavy load. There are a great many stressors that human beings are subject to. A few examples are cold, heat, drugs, poor diet, sorrow, illness, anger, and physical trauma. An exhaustive list would be near impossible.

It's pretty clear what stress is in a steel beam, but what exactly is stress in a human being?

**Stress Defined.**

Hans Selye has given the following definition of (*physiological*) *stress*: It's *the nonspecific response of the body to any kind of demand made on it (the demands being stressors).*

What exactly does *nonspecific* response mean? It's the essence of what stress means.

Stressors have *specific* effects; cold makes you shiver, a burn makes you blister, a physical injury may make you bruise or bleed, deep sorrow can make you weep, etc. Although stressors can be completely different, yet they all elicit essentially *the same biological response*. This is the non-specific response, the *stress*.

It's difficult to see how such different things such as cold, heat, drugs, illness, anger, sorrow and joy could all give an identical biochemical reaction in the body, never the less this is the case.

In a little more detail, a *stressor* is any demand on the body that requires the body to readjust or adapt in some way. *Any* demand does this, so any demand is a stressor. Stressors occur continually with various degrees of intensity all day, every day. It is relevant whether the agent or stimulation is pleasant or unpleasant, but the real health issue is in the intensity of the demand for readjustment or adaptation.

Stressors and the resulting stress-effects certainly can't completely be avoided; one is completely free of stress only with death! But here is a fact that makes stress such a confusing topic.

Some stressors and the resulting stress are *positive* and good for you, actually health-building! When someone is said to be "under stress" what is implied is the person is under *negative* stress, harmful stress is called *distress*. An even more confusing aspect of stress is that stressors can be processed differently by different persons. An example of this is two persons riding on a scary rollercoaster. The first person is frightened and holding on with white knuckles and can't wait for the ride to end, while the second person is exhilarated, smiling and enjoying a great time. Remember that too intense a stress, even an enjoyable one, can be dangerous.

Every disease causes a certain amount of stress, and *stress is involved in the development of every disease.*

## The Autonomic Nervous System

The effect of stress on the body can't be understood without some understanding of the body's *autonomic nervous system*. The term derives from the word "autonomous" meaning "acting on its own." So this is a part of your body that acts on its own. It has two major divisions: the *sympathetic* division and the *parasympathetic* division. The sympathetic division causes the body automatically without any consciously willed actions to respond to any stressor by increasing heart rate, blood pressure, air exchange volume, blood flow to muscles and all other functions needed to respond to the event at hand. Functions not essential at the moment to help with the situation that has caused the response are turned down or turned off. The body's response to stressors is extremely complex and we won't be going any further into this. We will later be discussing the adrenal glands which play a central role in stress.

The parasympathetic division of the autonomic nervous system, on the other hand, monitors body functions during times of rest, sleep, food digestion, and elimination, when the body is not in the stressful situation. The proper functioning of the autonomic nervous system is central in helping the body cope with stress.

As the many stressful situations occur in daily life, the sympathetic system is activated over and over again; often one can't dissipate the hyper-emergency state resulting from the repeated stimulations of the sympathetic nervous system. In this condition the heart rate may be speeded up, blood pressure may be increased, the stomach may tighten, and blood flow may be diverted from vital organs to increase nutrients to the muscles. These physiological changes are meant to be temporary and if not dissipated, the body is kept in this emergency state chronically and health is threatened. Being chronically stressed may lead to the autonomic nervous system losing its flexibility and no longer able to deal effectively with the accumulated stressful energy within the sympathetic nervous system.[2]

## What can we do about all this?

Fortunately there's a great deal we can do to protect ourselves from the damaging effects of stress and these can be divided into two categories: first, you may be able to remove or decrease the intensity of at least some stressors in your life, and secondly, you may be able to help your body cope with stress.

Here is a list of stressors (far from complete and with some overlaps) that you might be able to deal with and diminish:

A bad diet (too much sugar in the diet; too much alcohol; not enough nutritious food)
Not getting enough sleep or enough restful sleep
Bad air in your environment
A bad commute to work
Hate your job
In a bad marriage
Your children causing stress
Sickness is a serious stress
Radiation exposure
Drugs
Smoking
Bad digestion
Any health problem can be a stressor
Unhappy
Unfulfilled
Panic attacks
Sexual problems
Bullied

Except for removing negative stressors from your life, the single most important thing you can do to help your body fight the damaging effects of stress is to help the body cope. This we do by *making sure your regulation is not blocked* which is discussed below. This almost always will include the need to strengthen your adrenal glands. Since the adrenal glands play such an important role in the body's response to stress we will be begin by discussing them in some detail.

## The Adrenal Glands

The *adrenal glands* are two small glands that are located on top of the kidneys. There are two parts to the adrenals, the adrenal *medulla* and the adrenal *cortex*, and these have different functions. The medulla has many nerves coming from the sympathetic nervous system that can stimulate the production of epinephrine (adrenaline) and norepinephrine which then travel through the circulatory system to all parts of the body producing much of the stress response like speeding up the metabolism of cells, increasing blood pressure, dilating blood vessels to the heart while decreasing blood flow to organs not needed during times of stress, causing the liver to release glucose into the blood stream, dilating pupils, increasing muscle strength and mental activity, and dilating the brochials (this is why epinephrine is given during asthma attacks). An important hormone released by the cortex is *cortisol* which has important functions to perform also relating to the stress response, however, too much and excess levels over too long a time can be very damaging.

The adrenals have many roles besides those relating to the stress-response. For example, there is much evidence that if the adrenals are functioning properly, menopause will be more symptom-free. The adrenals also help with hormone balance after menopause.

I believe at least half of the adult population in the US has varying degrees of significant adrenal malfunction or exhaustion. This is almost always the result of too much stress not dissipated over too long a time resulting in decreased ability to cope properly. The result of this will always include loss of energy and less resistance to disease.

**Further Suggestions to Help the Body Cope:**

Here are a few hints that can be considered in helping cope with stress that go beyond what we've mentioned so far: A balanced exercise program (at least a regular program of walking); prayer; meditation; homeopathy can help; a good diet; being around positive people; and hobbies. Again this is a far from complete list.

**A Few Relaxation Techniques**

Sit comfortably and allow yourself to breath a little more slowly and a little more deeply. Close your eyes, it will close out some of the external stimulation. Breathe in through the nose and out through the mouth breathing deeply. Breathing deeply will give you greater relaxation, more oxygen coming in, and more clearance of carbon dioxide from the waste products of the body. Now let your belly go soft; being soft means you're breathing from the bottom part of your lungs which is desirable. If the muscles in your belly and abdomen relax, then all the other muscles in the body will relax. In through the nose and out through the mouth with the belly soft. To encourage this process you can say to yourself, "soft" as you breathe in and "belly" as you breathe out. If thoughts come, gently let them go and gently bring your mind back to "soft/belly". Now open your eyes and come back in the room. You can do this almost any time. This is the beginning of creating relaxation. It's an antidote to the stress-response, to the fight or flight response, to the tension in our muscles. It's a way of creating a relaxed state.[3]

Instead of sitting, it might be even better to lie on the floor on your back (hopefully there's a rug you can lay on). You then put your legs on a chair. Let me try to describe this more clearly: Your back is on the floor (rug), your knees are pointing straight up, and your lower legs and feet are resting on a chair. Your body is forming two right angles. This is a very relaxing position.

Then you can go for a walk, and instead of going the way we ordinarily go which is often times hurrying from one place to another, not paying much attention to what's going on, as you walk notice what you think and feel and hear. And just say to yourself, "car screeching to a halt, cold wind on my face." Walk with awareness. This also can create a state of relaxation.

Yoga, tai chi, and chi gong are also great for stress reduction. It would be too much to discuss these here.

Since the automatic stress-response is so destructive, it is obvious that nature meant it to be used in emergency situations only and these should occur infrequently. How many of today's chronically ill patients never escape the lion that is constantly chasing them? How many view the world as a fundamentally hostile place with suspicion and danger everywhere. Given that the stress-response can be initiated even by the perception of danger, it's possible that the stress-response can be operating ceaselessly with its benefits lost and only long-term destruction remaining.

## Getting Back from Our Detour into Stress

Getting back now to our client. If I find the client has blocked regulation, this I usually consider the first correction that needs attention. I believe that if a practitioner specializes in nothing more than just keep regulation open on all clients; this alone would make the practice worthwhile.

Later I'll give you some idea of the correction process we use if the client is blocked. The same process is used in most situations needing attention as they arise in the overall health assessment.

## Switched?

The next test could actually have been done first. It's called a test to determine if the client is *switched*. A practitioner will not have much success if a client is switched. Being switched was a concept introduced by George Goodheart into Applied Kinesiology from the earliest days. The test I use is not the same as that taught in AK, nor is the correction process the same.

So what does being switched mean? You can think of a subject being "switched" as being in a state where the information being processed by the physical body is unreliable. The person's circuits, so to speak, are crossed and the body is processing at least some information incorrectly. A state of dyslexia is part of being switched, but the concept goes beyond this.

The two previous tests (regulation blocked and switched) are considered preliminary and these need to be corrected before moving on with the assessment.

After the preliminaries have been attended to, I personally find that reflex most in need of attention and then determine if I can strengthen it on its own or are there other associated reflexes that need to be strengthened in order to properly help the most important one. Some of these associated reflexes, if they exist, may be in the form of what are called "causal chains" which are determined one after another (in a sequence). The associated reflexes must be strengthened in order to help that reflex most in need of help. The reflexes in a chain must be strengthened from the last reflex of the chain, then the next to the last, and so forth up toward the reflex the body indicated was most in need of attention. Often by attending to the associated reflexes, our main reflex usually gets all the help it needs.

# Endnotes

1. What I use for this purpose is Dr. Riftin's *Heart Variability Analysis*. See the reference in Appendix E.

2. The loss of flexibility is most likely identical to what we call blocked regulation.

3. This script and others are on the web-site: cmbm.org.

# Section 12: More on How We Strengthen a Reflex

When attending to any reflex in need of help, and this help applies to blocked regulation and being switched as well, there is a sequence of factors that need to be evaluated. Need I say that communicating with the body's intelligence through muscle-response testing is how all this is done?

(1) Is something you're eating contributing to the problem? A client may be intolerant to one or more foods, but it does not follow that these are major factors in a particular reflex that needs attention. But foods often are commonly significant factors in a physiological problem needing attention.

(2) Is there an infection that is part of the problem? Is there an immune challenge? Perhaps you have a bacteria infection? Perhaps you have a viral infection? Perhaps it's a parasitic infection?

(3) Are toxins involved? Here we have a very common factor. Perhaps the most common toxin we find as a relevant factor is mercury. Perhaps it is coming from the food chain? Very often its source is a person's dental fillings! Mercury is certainly not the only heavy metal common in our environment, lead, aluminum and cadmium are others (and not the only others).

(4) Are toxic chemicals involved? Perhaps formaldehyde out-gassing from new rugs or from pressed board furniture? Perhaps outgasing from dry cleaning? How about household cleaners containing ammonia or other dangerous solvents?

(5) Are dietary changes, some special nutritional supplements or herbal formulas needed? The answer here is almost always yes!

(6) Will homeopathy help?

(7) Are emotional factors involved?

(8) Are scars on the body involved? Here is an important blocking factor to health that is almost completely neglected by modern mainstream medicine. Scars can be very significant

factors that need to be evaluated. I'll say a little more about the important topic of scars in Appendix D.

There are even more factors that may be involved like something being worn (an electric watch, necklaces, ear rings, especially tongue or belly button rings). All the above factors are evaluated to determine what can be done to raise a suboptimal score on a reflex.

When what needs to be done is determined, I have the client work only on those reflexes associated with the most important reflex and this often does not involve the most important reflex itself. After correcting the underlying causes, and when the body is satisfied with the most important reflex - meaning that the score has gone to its optimal value - then we can determine what then is the next most important reflex to work on. In this way, from visit to visit, we can make progress toward optimal health. Of course, life-style changes may be needed to keep from returning a reflex score to a suboptimal level, and continuing support for a reflex whose score has been optimized may also be required.

There is another useful thing that I used to do, but which lately I've neglected. I used to have a new client fill out what's called a *symptom form*. The form has a comprehensive, organized listing of symptoms and the client is asked to indicate which ones are personally relevant and to estimate the intensity of discomfort of the symptom (0 to 4). The form is then assigned an overall score from the information supplied by the client. Then by having the client fill out the form again some months later, both the client and I can get another kind of indication of our progress. The overall score assigned to the form should be coming down. It's often the case that the client does not notice improvements that are slow but progressive, so this can be useful.

# Section 13: Some Typical Clinical Findings

*"When educated and innate intelligences are able to communicate with each other (a possibility which the not very distant future may disclose) we shall be able to make a correct diagnosis."*

*D. D. Palmer 1914*

From my experience here is a list of the most common weaknesses I see in the office:

## (1) Digestive Weakness

A healthy digestive system is certainly a requirement if you want to improve or keep your health. When your digestion is not as it should be, besides the fact that the body will not be properly nourished no matter how healthful the food you consume, improperly digested food will rot during its time in the gut and this not only can damage the intestines, but can be a major source of toxicity in the body. There is a great difference between properly digested food and rotted food in the gut! Visualize a piece of meat left in 98 degree heat (day and night) for a few days. It's not uncommon for such a mass (mess) to be distributed throughout your intestines on a regular basis. Toxins in the small intestines can cause inflammation in the delicate intestinal lining which can in turn cause what is called a "leaky gut." This is a common pathway by which toxins can get into the bloodstream by way of the gut causing much grief. Of course the inflammation itself is very dangerous and can lead to even more serious pathology in the gut. Another factor that should be mentioned here is *transit time*. This refers to the speed with which the fecal matter moves through the gut. Obviously the longer such a toxic mass is in the gut, the more severe the consequences. This is another important topic. So what to do about all this? Here are some suggestions:

A major cause of digestive problems is *not enough stomach acid and/or not enough digestive enzymes*. In my experience a large percentage of persons over forty years of age have digestive weakness to a significant degree. In fact, I would estimate 50% of the entire adult population in this country has digestive weakness. This percentage goes up with age and I would estimate 90% of everyone in this country over age 60 needs digestive help. Here's something that should surprise you: Just about all who thinks they have "acid indigestion" actually are not making enough digestive acid. I would estimate that for every ninety-nine persons who don't have enough stomach acid, there is *one* that has too much! This view is certainly at odds with what most persons think. Witness what I believe is the most unfortunate misinformation concerning digestion that we are presently exposed to, namely all the advertising we see on TV about antacids. The real problem is *too little acid*, not too much! What is considered an "acid stomach" is a stomach filled with fermentation caused by a *lack* of digestive power. In these situations, I mainly use a product called *Zypan®* by *Standard Process.* Certain enzymes in the stomach are activated only in a proper acid environment. Zypan is not only an acid replacement but it contains the needed enzymes also. It's of course always better to get your natural digestion working than to rely on something like Zypan, but you can't make progress toward improving your natural digestion with faulty digestion! There are of course other products that can be used besides Zypan,[1] and your more holistic health care practitioner should be able to advise you. One should be tested before using any of my suggestions (or anybody else's) even though there is little danger in anything I'm discussing. It's not always a bad idea if you can't find someone to test you to just try what you might be interested in and see if you feel better or worse. We recommend strongly that you go beyond the Zypan by adding a vegetable enzymes supplement and a pancreatic enzymes supplement to each meal.

For a stimulation, tonification and nourishing of the digestive system, which would require a little more patience to see results than by using something like Zypan, we recommend a *bitters herbal formula.* Just a small amount taken a few minutes before each meal can be extremely useful. It will also help turn-on the appetite, stimulate digestion and promote absorption and even elimination. Using a bitters formula is a great way to improve your health; it also can help regulate blood sugar, eliminate flatulence, and even help normalize liver function. Bitters are commonly used in other countries to aid digestion, e.g., you can find *Fernet* bitters (a good herbal product) in many Italian grocery stores.[2] We do not recommend any bitters product that contains a laxative ingredient. Laxatives should be used with great caution, if at all. Laxative dependence can be difficult to near impossible to correct.

**Checking for Digestive Weakness**

Placing my fingers just below the rib cage in the center of the body and the indicator going weak usually means weak digestive power in the stomach. About 90% of the time this weakness is corrected by a formula like *Zypan*. It's also very common to find NEC's with digestive weakness. Keep in mind that any weakness should be evaluated with a more detailed protocol in a setting of a collection of prioritized and perhaps associated weaknesses.

**(2) Adrenal Weakness**

There are three reflex areas on the body associated with the adrenals. I'm not sure at the moment if there are any differences between them; they seem redundant. One of these is just above the area of the kidneys on the client's back.[3] Weak adrenals are very common and there are many nutritional and herbal formulas that can strengthen them: Dr. Versendaal used a formula of nutrients called *Drenamin®* (from Standard Process) together with a combination of vitamin B6 and Niacinamide. An herbalist, whose opinion I value, recommends an herbal formula consisting of deglycerized Licorice Root and Rehmannia, and another excellent herbalist often uses the formula consisting of Eleuthro, Oat milky seed, Schesandra fruit, Gota Kola, Rhodiola root and American Ginseng. Then there is Vitamin C, and certain B complex factors (especially vitamin B5) that are very useful for the adrenals as well. There are almost always NEC's associated with adrenal weakness.

**(3) Mercury Toxicity**

This may be my most common finding, and I'm convinced that a good part of this is from the mercury fillings that most of you have in your teeth, but I also believe the sources of mercury pollution go well beyond this. This leads into the vast topic of detoxification which will not be discussed here to the extent it deserves. The two formulas I use to start a mercury detoxification are *Parotid®* and *Cholacol II®* (both from Standard Process). *Chlorella* (a sea algae) is also useful. I'm told that chlorella is the largest selling supplement in Japan; it seems to make users feel better. Can it be because it helps detoxify the mercury they consume in fish? The topic of detoxification from toxic metals, the most common being mercury, lead, aluminum and cadmium, is important and goes far beyond the little I've mentioned.

Other less common (but still common) weaknesses include *dysbiosis* (an unhealthy state of the gut), *parasite infestation* (more common than you might realize), *hormonal weaknesses, prostate weakness, sinus weakness, thyroid weakness, liver weakness, gallbladder weakness,* and *skin problems.* If, for example, a person has a skin rash, just touching a part of the affected skin causes an indicator to drop.

# Endnotes

1. Betaine HCL or Glutamic Acid HCL for example.

2. *Fernet* makes several products. The only one I recommend is the one with the formula consisting of: Aloe, quinine, gentian, rhubarb, zedoary, myrrh, chamomile, licorice, cardamom, galangai, centaury, imperatorial, angelica, calumba, saffron, and peppermint oil.

3. Adrenal literally means "above the kidneys."

# Section 13: Can anyone do this work?

Every so often I'll come across a person that I can't test no matter what I do to try and correct the situation. In the next section I'll list some of the ways one can try and establish the communication process if it's not working.

One important factor in being able to test is that the practitioner should be in good health. Being in poor health is a major reason for not being able to do muscle-response testing.

I believe the intelligence that is being accessed here will not reveal weaknesses that a person is completely unable to help. For example, a layperson may get feedback on the test to see if sugar weakens a person but perhaps not on a test for dysbiosis or for weak liver function.

Both the practitioner and client should be open to the communication interchange. If either does not want to be part of the testing process, it usually will not work.

Clients often tell me they went home and tried to do a muscle test on their spouse and they couldn't get a reaction. I would think the main reason would be the spouse considered it nonsense.

Not all persons are equally testable. Some require considerable experience on the part of the tester to get an interpretable response.

## Problems with Testing

I have little doubt that most practitioners who use muscle-response testing will at times not be able to get a response when testing a particular person. Some of my teachers seem never to have this problem; I've never seen Scott or Debbie Walker or Walter Melnicke ever find a patient that was not testable. Dr. Versendaal did occasionally find a patient who was not testable and his suggestion for solving this problem was generally to "adjust the ankles." I've tried to describe this adjustment in Appendix E. This suggestion does not often work for me.

All of my teachers are aware of the problem and do offer advice even though they themselves don't seem ever to experience it. I've collected a lengthy list of suggestions made by my teachers and colleagues on what one might try if experiencing this problem. I'm presenting just a sampling of these suggestions in the next section.

# Section 14: On Being Electrical

Dr. Versendaal speaks of a person being "electrical" or "not being very electrical." He says when the doctor is not sufficiently electrical, he or she won't be able to test very well. Likewise, if the patient is not very electrical, you may find the person untestable. Of course, the worst of all is when both the doctor and patient are not electrical.

Now what does "being electrical" or "not being electrical" mean? I think it has something to do with the size of the body's aura which I believe directly correlates to how healthy a person is. I mentioned that some practitioners never seem to have difficulty testing clients. I think this is due to the fact that they have strong "electricity." The more electrical one is the easier it is to test clients. If the patient is not testable, it's often the practitioner that is not electrical enough. So the only answer here is for the practitioner to work on building his or her own health.

We described how Dr. Anderson measured the size of a person's aura. Dr. Versendaal used a similar test to measure how electrical a person is. He would ask the person to hold out say the right hand (it could have been the left hand as well) palm down pointing the fingers out away from the body. While continuously testing an indicator muscle (the person's other arm), Dr. Versendaal would bring his hand toward the finger tips of the person's hand. The indicator would test strong until it got near the finger tips and then it would drop. How far Dr. Versendaal's hand got from the finger tips before the arm dropped indicated the intensity of the aura. Sometimes the indicator would not drop at all no matter how close to the finger tips Dr. Versendaal brought his hand. In this case the person had a very weak aura and probably was not testable.

In order to make the person more testable, Dr. Versendaal would invariably "adjust the ankles." If you want to test to see if the ankles need an adjustment you can do this by therapy localizing them. Dr. Versendaal would just point to the ankles while testing an indicator. Others may need to actually touch the ankles during the test. Adjusting a person's ankles often is very desirable independent of the question of testability. I've tried to describe this adjustment in Appendix F.

Dr. Anderson, you may recall, used the "figure-eights" procedure. If I want to make a subject more testable during an office visit, this is what I try first and it's the one I find most useful.

Finally, Dr. Versendaal told us that if none of these suggestions worked, "just put them on *the basic four* and have them return at a later time. He went on to say that this may take months to correct. He felt it was rarely needed. By "the Basic Four" he meant the Standard Process products: *For-Til B12®, B6 Niacinamide®, Catalyn®* and *Organic Iodine.* He said we could substitute Standard Process's *Min Tran®* for the Organic Iodine which I would recommend you do if using this suggestion, especially since the Organic Iodine (at least from Standard Process) is no longer available. I would suggest about six of each of the Basic Four per day with meals. This technique is actually building up the patient's health and the healthier the person, the more testable. There are of course many other ways of building health besides just taking the Basic Four. This technique is actually building up the patient's health, and the healthier the person, the more testable. There are of course many other ways of building health besides just taking the Basic Four.

I find that a good cervical adjustment (by a competent chiropractor) can make a person more electrical.

One should always be aware that a state of dehydration can make a person untestable. It's a good idea routinely to have a client drink some water before being tested.

If a person is not testable you might want to try some adrenal tonics, perhaps on yourself as well. We discussed some adrenal tonics earlier.

Emotional trauma can make a person less electrical. Emotional trauma a practitioner is going through or has recently gone through can make him or her unable to test.

Here's a suggestion form George Goodheart, the developer of Applied Kinesiology

"When patients who do not show clear therapy localization, it's usually because of the medications, drugs, they're taking. You may need to test them with RNA®, in their mouth." [Note: *RNA* is a product from *Standard Process.*]

I'll stop here but this is not the end of this topic.

# Section 15: We're all Connected

I actually haven't told you the most useful means I have of working with a client who I can't "communicate" with, one who I can't get any response using muscle-response testing. Before I tell you about this, I'm going to describe a demonstration that Dr. Versendaal sometimes demonstrates at his seminars. I think it's relevant here.

Picture Dr. Versendaal on the stage at one of his seminars and with him is a very sick person in a wheel chair. Dr. Versendaal points out a very healthy young fellow in the audience that clearly spends a lot of time in the gym and asks him to come up on the stage. Dr. Versendaal then demonstrates that the fellow's arm tests very strong. Now Dr. Versendaal puts a chair next to the patient in the wheel chair and asks the fellow to sit in the chair. After a minute or so Dr. Versendaal retests the young fellow's arm and it drops easily. Just being next to the sick person has weakened him.

There are many implications here. One of the less obvious (in fact quite remote) of these implications is this:

You have in your office two persons, one (person A) who needs to be evaluated but you can get no response in muscle-response testing. The second person (person B) is testing very well, that is, you can get clear responses in testing. What you can do, and what works extremely well, is you can use person B to test person A! You have them sit next to each other and you use person B's arm while you test reflexes on person A. It works perfectly and is in fact *the best technique I know to deal with a person I'm unable to test.*[1]

One immediate implication of all this is *we are all connected* in some amazing way.

# Endnotes

1. Some of us refer to this as "surrogate testing." I've been told it's illegal to use this term. It's apparently OK to use the term "indirect testing." Such a law doesn't make sense to me either.

# Section 16: How does one find such a practitioner?

The practitioner that is far and away the best referral for an assessment based on what is introduced in this book is Walter Melnicke. See Appendix E. Any good Applied Kinesiologist would at least come close to what I've discussed in the book.

Standard Process will refer you to a practitioner in your area that uses their products. Standard Process can be contacted by calling 1-800-848-5061

You can find practitioners that use Dr. Walker's NET by contacting his office (Appendix E).

There are far more AK chiropractors that use muscle-response testing then all other health care professionals combined. They very likely would not cover all I've discussed, but then again they would do much beyond what I've discussed. Unfortunately not all AK practitioners are equally skilled. Those that have passed the AK Diplomate exam would certainly be among the best. You can find an AK chiropractor by calling *the International College of Applied Kinesiology* (Appendix E).

In many parts of the country, finding a competent herbalist would probably not be easy. *The American Herbalist Guild* is a group of professional herbalists attempting to control the quality of their at the moment small profession. You can get a referral from the AHG by contacting them (Appendix E).

It was with Dr. Versendaal's *Contact Reflex Analysis* (CRA) that I first got started in this work. What he teaches is close to what I've discussed in this book.[1]

# Section 17: Some Final Thoughts

(1)

I said earlier that my practice can be considered as limited to raising reflex scores. But raising reflex scores means raising *health*. Here are some wonderful statements that sum up a main message implied of this book:

*Disease tends to disappear in the presence of health.*


*You're not sick because you have a disease;*
*You have a disease because you're sick.*

(2)

Before we come to the end, a few more thoughts on exactly who or what we're communicating with during a muscle-response testing procedure. The following is from David Hawkins's book *Power Versus Force*:

*Yet we cannot even locate the source of this intelligence. We have said where it is not: residing in the human consciousness. ...*
*Does it emanate down from an external God to men? ... Does it emanate out from the God that is within the center of man's being?*

I mentioned earlier that as far as I know muscle-response testing has been completely unknown throughout human history. Perhaps this is not quite true. There is certainly the possibility that the same communication we experience may be obtained by means other than muscle-response testing. For example, does this relate to the work of Edgar Casey?[1] Do oriental mystics or shamans use facilities that are equivalent to muscle-response testing? Perhaps sometime in the distant past this phenomenon actually was discovered, and since it was so clear that there was a communication with a higher intelligence, perhaps this resulted in the concept of a guardian angel.

No matter what future developments may bring, one thing is certain to me, the process of muscle-response testing should be approached with great respect and reverence. [2]

# Endnotes

1. See, for example, edgarcasey.com

2. For a deep discussion of the concept of Reverence, you might want to read Professor Woodruff's book listed in the section on Relevant Books and Papers.

# Appendix A: Sugar

"Sugar has been blamed for every known disease, and while these accusations may sound like exaggerations, they are closer to the truth than you might realize.

The far-reaching problems sugar can cause are documented in medical journals throughout the world and more sugar-disease connections are found each year.

This information never found its way to the general public, and even the little there was got lost in all the outcries about the evils of fat. Americans ended up blaming fat for their health problems instead of sugar, and since then health problems have gotten worse."

(Louise Gittleman)

Here is a list of diseases that have a sugar-related component:

Acne; Addiction to drugs, caffeine and food; Adrenal gland exhaustion; Alcoholism; Allergies; Anxiety; Appendicitis; Arthritis; Asthma; Behavioral problems; Binge eating; Bloating; Bone loss; Cancer (particularly breast, colon and rectal cancers); Candidiasis; Cataracts; Colitis; Constipation; Depression; Dermatitis; Diabetes; Difficulty concentrating; Diverticulitis and diverticulosis; Eczema; Edema; Emotional problems; Endocrine gland dysfunction; Fatigue; Food cravings; Gallstones; Gout; Heart disease; High blood cholesterol; High estrogen levels; High triglyceride levels; Hormone problems; Hyperactivity; Hypertension; Hypoglycemia; Impaired digestion; Indigestion; Insomnia; Kidney stones; Liver dysfunction; Liver enlargement and fatty liver syndrome; Low HDL cholesterol; Menstrual difficulties; Mental illness; Mood swings; Muscle pain; Nearsightedness; Obesity; Osteoporosis; Overacidity; Parasitic infections; Premature aging and wrinkles; Premenstrual syndrome; Psoriasis; Rheumatism; Shortened life-span; Tooth decay; Ulcers; Vaginal yeast infections; Weakened immunity.

Our bodies do not need simple sugars at all. We get all the sugar we need from a good diet. We can live perfectly well on vegetables, fruits, legumes and grains. Here's an estimate of average sugar intake over the years in our country:

| Year | Amount in Pounds |
|------|------------------|
| Early 1800's | 12 |
| 1850 | 22 |
| 1875 | 41 |
| 1895 | 63 |
| 1915 | 95 |
| 1935 | 115 |
| 1955 | 119 |
| 1976 | 125 |
| 1990 | 130-140 |

# Appendix B: Aspartame (also known as NutriSweet® or Equal®)

"I don't want my child or myself consuming all that sugar, so I switched to NutraSweet." Why not? Ten's of millions of Americans have said they don't want white table sugar, corn syrup or fructose, but they want their things sweet. They're told this is a natural sweetener and it's even non-caloric.

Jim Turner Esq. (one of the original *Nader's Raiders*) author of the book *The Chemical Feast*, in 1980 filed the first legal objections to aspartame, and persuaded the FDA to conduct a public board of inquiry into the safety of the substance. This public board ruled unanimously that aspartame should not be marketed because of the possibility it might cause brain tumors. *However, an FDA Commissioner overruled the public board's decision.* Mr. Turner subsequently helped to uncover data showing a 10% rise in brain tumors following the introduction of aspartame into the market.

NutriSweet and Equal are the most well-known names in the US for aspartame. It's a combination of two amino acids: aspartic acid and phenylalanine that are bound using methyl alcohol. The problem is that two of these three substances are clearly neurotoxins and the third can be a serious problem for some. Phenylalanine can cause a disorder called *phenylketonuria*, and every child is tested for this at birth. There may be as many as 30,000 who have this phenylketonuria problem. Then aspartic acid is known to cause lesions in the brains of mice, and methyl alcohol (wood alcohol) is a poison known to cause a whole series of problems including blindness or even death. The industry argument is that the amount of methyl alcohol present in NutriSweet is so small, and much smaller than the amounts that cause blindness and death, and therefore should be considered safe. But does a small amount of a toxin mean it's safe for all? And keep in mind aspartame is in about 5,000 food products. We know that aspartic acid in animal studies does cause little holes in the brain at very small amounts that are comparable to what persons do consume. Basically what we're being told is that a small hole in the brain is not really a serious problem. Maybe that's true just once? But what if you do it every day for years?

97

It's a little wonder we have over 10,000 complaints to the FDA from people who have had serious seizures, headaches, impaired vision, hives, neurological hives, and epileptic seizures. Incidentally, all of the animal studies on NutriSweet showed high-doses caused epileptic seizures. The whole picture is one of a very serious toxin that has been put into the public's food supply by political pressure.

# <u>Appendix C: Gluten</u>[1]

Gluten is actually a family of proteins found mainly in wheat, but also in lesser amounts in oats and rye. It's also present in small amounts in some lesser known grains. Celiac disease which has been known to establishment medicine for at least fifty years is an ailment where the inside layer of the small intestine is chronically damaged by gluten proteins and by its interaction with the immune system. Celiac disease should be considered the most severe cases of the more general class of gluten sensitivity. Until recently celiac disease was considered rare. Instead of the one in about five thousand which was the estimate up until about ten years ago, it is now estimated to be about one in one hundred! Undiagnosed and of course untreated celiac disease has been implicated in many diseases including cancer, autoimmune diseases, neurological diseases, chronic pain syndromes, psychiatric disorders and other brain disorders, and premature death. There is also evidence linking it to some cases at least of osteoporosis, epilepsy, ADD and other learning disorders, chronic liver disorders and even short stature. Yet it is estimated that only one case of celiac disease in every forty is ever diagnosed! As I mentioned celiac disease is only a small part (but a severe part) of a much large group: the gluten sensitive. With about 1 % of the US population suffering from celiac disease, about 1/3rd of the US population is gluten sensitive![2] Gluten sensitivity is diagnosed even less often (much less often) that celiac disease. Gluten sensitivity has also been linked to a long list of disorders of "unknown origin." Gluten sensitivity usually accompanied by nutritional deficiencies and can result in a great number of health problems.

1. This information has been extracted from Dr. James Braly's book: *Dangerous Grains*, Avery, 2002.

2. Of course the problem extends far beyond the US alone. I believe it is a world-wide epidemic.

# **Appendix D: Scars**

Traditional Chinese medicine has always taught that cutting any part of the body is very undesirable to say the least. "Shame on you if you need an operation; you should have practiced better prevention." Of course some operations can't be prevented, but the point is they can do serious damage. What they have in mind is the cutting through an energy meridian which they believe will impede the flow of Qi.

When trying to determine the causes of a reflex that test weak, we often find scars to be significant factors. Here's a good example. Many women have an episiotomy scar. This is on the conception vessel (a meridian we spoke of above). Also on the conception vessel is the thyroid! Is this at least part of the reason for so much Synthroid® being prescribed?

Any scar, no matter how small, can be a factor in bringing down your health. On the other hand, a scar may be of little or no consequence. So let's say you have a scar that is significant; can anything be done? The answer is yes, a lot can be done. I'm told that after an operation scars are routinely treated in Germany.

There are three approaches that I'm aware of to treat a scar. I've many times verified (using muscle-response testing) the effectiveness of two of these. The first and easiest way to treat a scar is to rub wheat germ oil into the scar once or twice a day. It may take a month or more before the scar no longer indicates as a factor in whatever it originally was found to be. The second method is to use a cold laser on the scar. The light is shined on the scar for about four minutes per treatment. The number of treatments will of course vary with the case. The third method is much more costly and can be done only by a licensed medical doctor that is trained in the technique (there are very few of these around). The technique involves injections into the scar. I have had no experience with this so far.

# Appendix E

**Standard Process Labs**

1200 West Royal Lee Drive, Palmyra, WI 53156-0904

(800)-848-5061

They will refer you to a practitioner in your area that uses their products. This is not an unreasonable way to find a practitioner that knows something about nutrition.

**Walter Melnicke, Ph.D.**

New York City

212-989-0928

**Scott and Debbie Walker**

They offer several educational programs on their Neuro-Emotional work. I highly recommend that any health care professional take at least their Basic Seminar.

They can be contacted at: NET Inc. 510 Second Street, Encinitas, CA 92024. Their phone is 760-944-1030.

**The International College of Applied Kinesiology**

6405 Metcalf Avenue, Suite 503, Shawnee Mission, Kansas, 66202

Phone: 913-384-5336

**Eugene Charles** DC, DIBAK *Applied Kinesiology in Clinical Practice: The 100 Hour Course.* My hope is that someday every chiropractor will be proficient in AK. This course is the best way I know of getting started.

**The American Herbalist Guild**
1931 Gaddis Road
Canton, GA 30115
(770)-751-6021


**John Diamond MD** PO Box 381 South Salem NY 10590

His weekend seminars have been offered four times a year. He also
has several books, all relevant to our topic. I've listed a few of these
below.

**Alexander Riftin PhD**
Heart Rhythm Instruments, Inc.
173 Essex Ave
Metuchen, NJ 08840
www.NervExpress.com
(732)-635-1144


**Wendell Whitman** *Trinity School of Natural Health*, Winona Lake,
IN.

**Wendell W. Whitman M.Div**
401 Kings Highway
Winona Lake, Indiana 46590
1-800-428-0408

**D. A. Versendaal D.C., Ph.D.**
1-214-438-6932

# Appendix F: Dr. Versendaal's Ankle Adjustment

Six major energy meridians flow through the ankles. If this flow is impeded, the energy to the *upper* part of the body will be lessened which can lead to gradual deterioration of, e.g., hearing, eyesight, and even the health of the hair.

Ankles that need an adjustment can also cause a weakening of *all* the muscles of the body (including, e.g., the heart!). Another consequence of this problem is that chiropractic adjustments in general won't hold as well as they should. (For this latter problem, the uterous or prostate reflex must also be strong.)

It's easy to show you "live" how to adjust an ankle, and I'm happy to show you at any time. Here I'll try to describe the procedure to you in words.

There are many ways of doing the adjustment:

(1) With shoes off (sox on is OK), sit down and bring your left ankle on top of your right knee. Now grab the top of your left foot (just above the left toes) with your right hand. Your left hand can hold onto your left ankle. Now with your right hand, pull the left foot down sharply. You are trying to open the joint inside the ankle, between the foot and the lower leg. You are pulling down so the foot is going into a position like a ballerina would be in if she were standing on her toes. Then you should repeat the same movement with your hand rotated slightly toward the direction of the small toe. Then repeat it one last time with the hand rotated toward the big toe. It is very desirable to hear a snapping sound when you pull down. There is almost no chance of hurting yourself by doing this. Finally, do the same with the other foot, i.e., your right ankle is put on top of your left knee and you repeat all the above adjustments.

Here is another way of doing the adjustment. You're standing this time.

(2) Take off your shoes (sox on is find). Place the top of your right foot on the seat of a chair. Your right heel is pointing up. Place your right hand on this heel and press down sharply.

# Some Relevant Books and Papers

Benson, Herbert, MD. *The Relaxation Response*, Harpertorch, 1975.

Diamond, John MD.
- *Your Body Doesn't Lie*, Warner Books, 1979.
- *Life Energy*, Paragon House, NY, 1990.
- *The Collected Papers of John Diamond MD: Volume I and Volume II*. The Diamond Center, LLC, 1980, PO Box 381, South Salem, NY 10590
- *Life-Energy Analysis: A Way to Cantillation*, Archaeus Press, Valley Cottage, NY, 1988.

Erdman, Robert.
- *The Amino Revolution*, Century Books, 1987.
- *Fats That Can Save Your Life*, Progressive Health Publishing, 1990.

Kenndle and Kenndle. Muscles: Testing and Function, Baltimore: Williams & Wilkins, 2nd Edition, 1971.

*Hawkins, David MD. Power versus Force,* Hay House, Inc. 1995.

International Journal of Neuroscience, a 1989 article is on muscle-response testing.

Nambudripad, Devi S. MD DC L.Ac., Ph.D. *Say Good-Bye To Illness: A Revolutionary Treatment for Allergies and Allergy-Related Conditions*, Third Edition, Delta Publishing Company.

Monti, Daniel MD et al. Muscle Test Comparisons of Congruent and Incongruent Self-Referential Statements, *Perceptual and Motor Skills*, 1999, 88, 1019-1028.

Reich, Wilhelm MD. His life and work is fascinating. He was involved in many different fields of research, and in the latter part of his career he seemed to rediscover Qi (he called it *Orgone energy*) and he performed many incredible experiments on it. He wrote several books that may not be easy reading, but they're all worthwhile. Our government agencies persecuted him (mainly for his application of orgone energy to cancer patients.) He died in prison in 1953.

Sapolsky, Robert. *Why Zebras Don't Get Ulcers*, W. H. Freeman and Company, 1998.

Selye, Hans. *The Stress of Life*, A Signet Book, 1974.

- *Stress Without Distress*, New American Library, 1974.

Lee, Miriam, OMD. *Insights of a Senior Acupuncturist*, Blue Poppy Press, 1992.

Riftin, Alexander. *Nerve-Express: System Guide and User's Manual*, Heart Rhythm Instruments, Inc. 173 Essex Avenue, Metuchen, NJ 08840 www.nerveexpress.com. This manual describes a piece of equipment every health care practice should investigate.

Vithoulkas, George. *The Science of Homeopathy*. Grove Weidenfeld, NY 1980. (For a more introductory treatment of Homeopathy, you might rather read another of his books:
*Homeopathy: Medicine for the New Man*, Arco Publishing, New York, 1979.)

Walther, David S. *Applied Kinesiology: Synopsis*. SDC Systems DC, 275 West Abriendo Aveenue, Pueblo, Colorado 81004. (This book is intended for professionals. I don't know of a book on Applied Kinesiology I would recommend for the general reader.)

Weiss, Rudolf Fritz MD. *Herbal Medicine*, (Translated from the Sixth German Edition), Beaconsfield Publishers, LTD, England, 1988.

Mills, Simon and Bone, Kerry. *Principles and Practice of Phytotherapy: Modern Herbal Medicine.* Churchill Livingston, 2000.

Lee, Royal. - *The Therapeutic Manual*, Standard Process Labs, Palmyra, WI.
- *The Product Bulletin*, Standard Process labs.
- *Lectures of Royal Lee: Volume I*, Selene River Press, 1998.

Dr. D. A. Versendaal. *Contact Reflex Analysis: A Physician's Desk Reference for Alternative Health Care*, Hoezee Manufacturing, 1993.

Woodruff, Paul. *Reverence: Renewing a Forgotten Virtue*, Oxford University Press, 2001.

# Some Acknowledgements

**Royal Lee**: Founder of Standard Process Labs, and in my opinion, number one among persons that have made the most important contributions to the field of applied nutrition.

**Gary Null**: The person whose teachings on health issues I most value.
.
**D.A. Versendaal**: One of the pioneers in this work and the person who first introduced me to muscle-response testing and who got me started in this work.

**Walter Melnicke**: My friend and in my opinion the best practitioner I know in the applications of muscle-response testing.

**David Winston:** He offers a two-year professional program in Herbal Medicine. I've taken the program and it's excellent and I recommend it to any health care professional.

**Bernard Jensen**: I had the good fortune to have studied with him. His teachings on nutrition are first rate. Every one of his numerous books is worth reading.

**John Lindseth**: I'm a graduate of his *School of Classical Taoist Herbology*. It was a wonderful program. Unfortunately he is no longer with us.

**Eugene Charles:** Offers a 100-Hour course in Applied Kinesiology, extremely valuable and interesting. My hope is that some day every chiropractor will be proficient in this.

**Heriberto Gonzales ND**: He got me started in the health field with his *School of the Naturopathic Health Sciences.*

**Carlton Fredericks**: I was a devoted listener to the last twenty-five years of his radio program which ran for about fifty years. He also is no longer with us. He got me interested in health and nutrition.

**Kerry Bone**: One of the most prominent herbal scientists today. I'm also a graduate of his professional program in herbal medicine.

**Robert Stewart**: I'm a graduate of his *School of Classical Homeopathy.*

**Wendell Whitman**: I've taken many of his courses, all of considerable value, on a variety of health topics. His address and phone number is listed above in case you're interested in being a student in one of his programs.

**Donald Warren DDS**: His seminars on the applications of muscle-response testing are excellent. He includes in these seminars the little-known, very important role your teeth play in your health, a role almost completely unknown in mainstream medicine. This is a topic I did not discuss in this book.

**Daniel Gole DDS**: I hope he is still giving seminars. Here you will find the complete story of how your teeth play such an important role in your overall health.

**Herbert Anderson DC**: I attended his monthly Applied Kinesiology lectures for the last four years of his life. Unfortunately I missed the first twenty years of these lectures.